Dr Philippa Kaye MBBS (Hons), MA (Hons) (Cantab), MRCGP, DCH, DRCOG, DFSRH is a young GP who trained at Downing College, Cambridge, followed by Guy's, King's & St Thomas' medical school. She is the author of *The Fertility Handbook* and *Coping with Diabetes in Childhood & Adolescence* and has a regular column in *Junior* magazine. She lives in London with her husband and son.

To my husband Ben, for holding my hand and heart throughout my pregnancy and beyond, and our wonderful son Harrison who makes me happier than I ever thought possible.

YOUR PREGNANCY
Week by Week

Dr Philippa Kaye

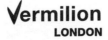
LONDON

1 3 5 7 9 10 8 6 4 2

Published in 2010 by Vermilion, an imprint of Ebury Publishing

Ebury Publishing is a Random House Group company

Copyright © Philippa Kaye 2010

Philippa Kaye has asserted her right to be identified as the author of this work in accordance with the Copyright, Designs and Patents Act 1988.

The Random House Group Limited Reg. No. 954009

Addresses for companies within the Random House Group can be found at www.rbooks.co.uk

A CIP catalogue record for this book is available from the British Library

The Random House Group Limited supports The Forest Stewardship Council (FSC), the leading international forest certification organisation. All our titles that are printed on Greenpeace approved FSC certified paper carry the FSC logo. Our paper procurement policy can be found at www.rbooks.co.uk/environment

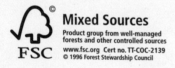

Mixed Sources
Product group from well-managed forests and other controlled sources
www.fsc.org Cert no. TT-COC-2139
© 1996 Forest Stewardship Council

FSC

Printed and bound in Great Britain by Clays Ltd, St Ives Plc

Illustrations by Dave Williams @ The Apple Agency Ltd

ISBN 9780091929305

Copies are available at special rates for bulk orders. Contact the sales development team on 020 7840 8487 for more information.

To buy books by your favourite authors and register for offers, visit www.rbooks.co.uk

contents

acknowledgements

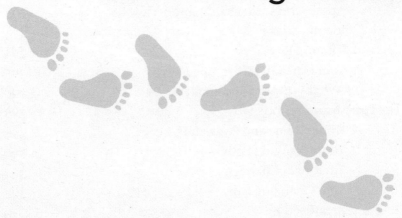

I would like to thank Vibha Ruparelia, consultant obstetrician at the Whittington Hospital, for her help and guidance regarding obstetrics and checking the book for errors!

Thanks to Becky Mallison for checking the yoga sections in the book.

Thanks must also be given to Julia Kellaway, my editor at Vermilion, for her direction and valuable comments on the manuscript, and to my agent, Jane Graham Maw, for her support and for seeing my potential.

Although I have been taught by many fantastic doctors and teachers, I owe a debt of gratitude to my GP trainer, Dr Amanda Sutton, for her wise teaching, counsel and friendship.

Thanks, too, as always, to my family: my husband, parents, siblings and more, for their steadfast support and assistance in all I do. Without all of them I would be lost.

introduction

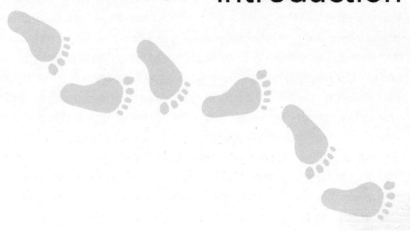

Pregnancy is an extremely exciting time. As your body changes and your baby grows and develops inside you, you will already be on the path to becoming a parent. You are likely to have lots of questions, not only about what is happening to your body and your baby but also about planning for the future, for labour itself and for life with a baby afterwards. When I was pregnant, every twinge or symptom sent me running for my medical textbooks until my husband threatened to confiscate them!

I feel that the best way to enjoy your pregnancy and prepare for labour and the challenges and joys of parenthood is to be informed about your options. This will help you make educated choices for yourself and your baby. Some women, like me, want to know as much as possible, while others find that too much information can make them unnecessarily anxious. Most women will probably pick a middle course, finding out as much as they feel comfortable with, and you will choose what is right for you. Each pregnancy can be different and raise new questions, so whether this is your first pregnancy or second, third, fourth or more, I hope you will find the answers in this book. Remember, though, you should always talk to your antenatal team if you have any concerns.

This book takes you through your pregnancy week by week, explaining what is happening to your baby and body. The exact times of a baby's development are not yet known, so you may find that certain times in this book are different from those mentioned in others. Your baby, whether it will be a girl or a boy, is referred to as 'he' throughout the book to make it easy to differentiate from you, as a 'she'. The changes occurring to your body have been separated out into individual weeks, though in reality the changes are more fluid and can occur concurrently. Each week also describes and explains a common symptom of pregnancy, such as morning sickness or indigestion, and gives advice on how to help relieve it, if possible, and when to see your doctor. Again, though, there is no hard-and-fast rule as to when these symptoms will present themselves; you can get the symptoms or conditions described either earlier or later than mentioned in the book. The book focuses on a normal pregnancy, and any common symptoms or issues that arise. If there are any complications in your pregnancy, your antenatal team will be able to discuss them in more detail with you, though remember the majority of pregnancies are uncomplicated and healthy!

Each week also has a section on lifestyle – generally diet, exercise or sex as pregnant women often have questions about these areas. Some weeks also have a section on yoga, describing breathing techniques and some simple yoga poses which are safe in pregnancy, to help keep you strong, supple and flexible and may even help with backache! As you go through your pregnancy you will have various antenatal appointments and tests; these are all described at the relevant times. Common concerns and practical elements, such as what to buy for baby, are also covered. The section on labour describes all the options that you may have, as well as the process of labour. Finally, there is a chapter on the first six weeks after delivery, the 'postpartum period'. Throughout the book there are sections aimed at expectant dads called 'For fathers', so get them to have a read too; this will help keep them involved in the pregnancy and the process of becoming a father. On pages 322–323 you will find a timeline of your pregnancy and the structure of the standard antenatal care for your reference.

Although I have tried to explain the complicated and intricate process of pregnancy in simple, understandable language, I have used some medical terms within the text. Each of these will be explained, and there is also a Glossary at the back of the book for you to refer to. You will be hearing some medical terms from your doctor and midwife, and it helps to know what they are talking about! Some of the terms may appear quite cold. For example, the developing baby is called an embryo or foetus, while you think of it simply as your baby.

Another thing you'll need to understand is the concept of 'trimesters'. Pregnancy is divided into three sections, or trimesters, though there are differences of opinion as to the exact cut-off point of each trimester. The first trimester is the first 12 or 13 weeks of your pregnancy and is the time in which all your baby's organs and bones develop. The second trimester is between Weeks 13 and 26 of pregnancy. In this time the baby continues to develop and mature, and you will begin to feel the baby's movements. The third trimester lasts approximately from Week 27 until the end of pregnancy, Week 40, and is the time in which the baby grows, putting on weight and maturing in preparation for labour and life after birth.

I hope you find this book a useful companion during your pregnancy – not just for yourself but for your partner too. You may choose to read the book all the way through, or as you enter each week; alternatively you may choose to dip in and out, to check something, to read about a symptom or to find out what your baby is doing this week. Whatever you choose to do, I hope you find the book easy to understand, informative and helpful as you go through your pregnancy and enter parenthood.

weeks 1–4

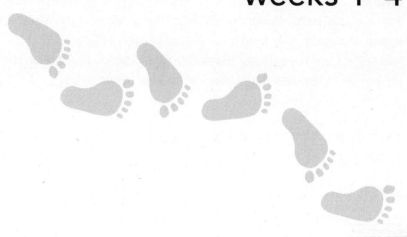

Women are pregnant for nine months ... for 40 weeks or 280 days, which is actually just over nine calendar months. However, you are actually pregnant for only 38 weeks, and only know that you are for approximately 36 weeks! This is because during what doctors call the first few weeks of your pregnancy conception has not yet occurred.

It can be confusing but remember that the first day of your period is the first day of your menstrual cycle, and is considered to be the first day of Week 1. The average woman will then ovulate at around day 14 of her menstrual cycle, so at the end of Week 2. If you are going to become pregnant, conception occurs within a few days of ovulation; although you are then 'pregnant', you will not be aware of it. The average woman has a 28-day cycle, and so becomes aware of a late period at around the end of the fourth week, or approximately two weeks after conception. If you normally have a longer cycle, say five weeks, you would not be aware of any pregnancy until later.

When your period is late you may do a pregnancy test. How many weeks pregnant you are is calculated from the date of the first day of your last period (this date is defined as the last menstrual period or LMP). So you may have been aware of the fact that you are pregnant for only five minutes but it will have been approximately two weeks since conception, and your doctor will say you are about four weeks pregnant already! Although you wouldn't be able to see your baby on a scan at this stage, your baby will have the genes of a boy or girl, or you may already have twins. All the information about eye colour, hair colour and many other characteristics is already encoded in the genes within the cells that will make up your baby.

THE MENSTRUAL CYCLE AND CONCEPTION

Week 1

The menstrual cycle and therefore Week 1 starts on the first day of your period, which lasts approximately five to seven days. The 'blood' shed is a combination of the lining of your womb (endometrium) and blood. The hormone changes that stimulate your period to start also stimulate the brain to produce luteinising hormone (LH) and follicle stimulating hormone (FSH).

Week 2

As the levels of LH and FSH rise, they stimulate the production of follicles within the ovary. These are fluid-filled sacs containing eggs. Although approximately 20 follicles start to grow in each cycle, usually only one will become larger than the others, and will be the follicle to produce the egg. The developing follicle begins to produce the hormone oestrogen, which stimulates the lining of the womb to become thick so implantation can occur. At approximately day 14, at the end of Week 2 or beginning of Week 3 of your cycle, ovulation occurs. Rising oestrogen levels stimulate the brain to produce a short sharp burst, or peak, of LH. Ovulation occurs 24–36 hours later when an egg is released from the follicle and is picked up by the fimbriae, or tendrils, at the end of the fallopian tubes. It is transported into the fallopian tubes to begin to travel into the womb.

Around the time of ovulation, oestrogen acts on the cervical mucus produced by the woman to make it thin and watery so it is easy for sperm to travel through it, through the cervix (neck of the womb) and into the womb. During intercourse, at the point of ejaculation, sperm are released in the semen into the vagina. They travel though the cervix, into the womb and then up to the fallopian tubes to potentially fertilise an egg.

Week 3

An egg needs to be fertilised within approximately 24 hours of ovulation or it begins to break down. Sperm, however, can survive for a few days while waiting to fertilise an egg. Fertilisation generally takes place in the fallopian tube and is the process by which one singular sperm enters the egg. Humans have 46 chromosomes in each of their cells, apart from in eggs or sperm; these contain only 23 chromosomes. When the sperm enters the egg, fertilisation occurs and a cell with 46 chromosomes is produced.

From this point onwards, this one cell has the potential to turn into a baby. The cell begins to divide and replicate and is now called a zygote. The zygote travels down the fallopian tube into the womb, a journey that takes three to four days, with the cells multiplying all the time. Once in the womb, the zygote remains there for a few days before implantation occurs.

During this time, the shell the egg comes from (now called the corpus luteum) produces the hormone progesterone and small amounts of oestrogen. Progesterone acts on the now thickened lining of the womb to prepare it for implantation of a fertilised egg. It also stimulates the endometrium to secrete a substance to help nourish the fertilised egg. This process occurs even if fertilisation has not taken place.

Week 4

Implantation is the process by which the fertilised egg inserts itself into the endometrium, or lining of the womb. This generally occurs five to seven days after fertilisation. Some women describe a cramping sensation or even a sharp discomfort around this time, which they attribute to implantation, and some women report some very light spotting.

Once implanted, the cells continue to divide. As they become more developed the zygote is called a blastocyst; these cells will form the placenta, membranes and baby. The site of implantation determines where your placenta will form. In the early stages of pregnancy

HOW DO TWINS OCCUR?

Multiple pregnancies, be they twins, triplets or more, occur in one of two ways. More than one egg may be released: two eggs, for example, may be fertilised by different sperm. This will result in non-identical twins as the babies come from different eggs and sperm, and therefore have a different genetic structure. Each baby will have its own placenta, umbilical cord and membranes. Alternatively, one egg may be released and fertilised with one sperm as with a single pregnancy; however, for reasons as yet unknown, the zygote splits into two separate zygotes which will become twins. In this case the twins will be identical as they share the same genes. Identical twins may share a placenta but each has an umbilical cord. Non-identical twins run in families, though identical twins do not. Multiple pregnancies are more common in older women (as they are more likely to release more than one egg) and in those taking fertility drugs which encourage the ovaries to release more than one egg.

the baby is referred to as the 'embryo'; after eight weeks of pregnancy, it is called the 'foetus'.

By the end of Week 4 the cells have become specialised enough to secrete the hormone beta human chorionic gonadotrophin (βHCG or HCG). This is the hormone that, among other actions, will turn your pregnancy test positive. At the end of the fourth week of your menstrual cycle you would usually expect your period; if you are pregnant you will soon find out. If you were to do a transvaginal ultrasound scan, a gestational sac may already be seen within your womb (though this may not be seen until the end of Week 5). This sac contains the embryo, which as yet cannot be seen. Your womb starts off about the size of a plum or pear and increases in size to cover more of your abdomen in pregnancy.

If fertilisation does not occur, the levels of the hormones oestrogen and progesterone begin to fall, triggering the shedding of the endometrium, your period. This then triggers the cycle to start again.

Boy or girl?

Every cell in your body (apart from eggs and sperm) contains 46 chromosomes, made up of 23 pairs. Of these, the last pair, chromosomes 45 and 46, are the sex chromosomes. If you have the chromosomes XX you are female, and the chromosomes XY mean you are male. Eggs and

$$\text{X} + \text{X} = \text{XX}$$

Girl

$$\text{X} + \text{Y} = \text{XY}$$

Boy

sperm each contain only 23 chromosomes, one of each chromosome. All eggs contain one copy of the X chromosome; however, sperm can contain either the X or Y chromosome. Therefore it is the sperm (or the father) that determines the sex of the baby. An X sperm meeting an X egg makes an XX embryo, which will be a girl. A Y sperm meeting an X egg makes an XY embryo, which will be a boy. There are various theories about how to ensure you have a boy or a girl, from the food you eat to the timing of when you have sex (the theory being that Y sperm swim faster but X sperm live longer). However, in reality, the odds of you having a boy or a girl are about 50:50.

TAKING VITAMINS BEFORE AND DURING PREGNANCY

It is recommended that all women who are trying to conceive or who are pregnant should take folic acid supplements. Folic acid is a B vitamin found naturally in foods such as leafy vegetables like broccoli or spinach, and in beans and lentils, and is often added to fortified cereals. Taking supplements of folic acid in pregnancy has been shown to decrease the risk of conditions such as spina bifida, which can result in severe disabilities to the child. You should take 400 micrograms (mcg) per day up to 13 weeks' gestation. Some mothers may be advised by their doctors to take a higher dose of 5mg, for example if you are diabetic, have epilepsy or have had a previous child affected by spina bifida.

It is also important to keep up your vitamin D stores during pregnancy. Vitamin D is formed in our bodies after sun exposure on our skin, and is also found in foods such as oily fish and fortified cereals. Certain groups of women are more likely to have low vitamin D levels: women whose diet is low in vitamin D, such as vegans; women who have very limited sunlight exposure; women of African, Caribbean, Middle Eastern or South Asian origin; and women who are overweight (body mass index over 30). It is recommended that you take a supplement containing 10mcg of vitamin D per day throughout your pregnancy and if you are breastfeeding, especially if you are in a high-risk group as described above.

Both folic acid and vitamin D supplements can be bought over the counter at your supermarket or pharmacy. They can also be obtained as part of a 'pregnancy multivitamin'. You may be eligible to receive free vitamins as part of the Healthy Start programme (for more information see page 131).

You should aim to eat a varied diet containing all the major food groups, such as proteins, carbohydrates and fats with lots of fruit and vegetables (for more information see page 36). If you have a good diet you shouldn't need to take any other vitamin supplements. Some women, such as vegans (for more information see page 84), may be advised by their doctor to take vitamin supplements.

PREGNANCY TESTS

When the fertilised egg implants in the wall of your womb, the very young and developing placenta begins to secrete the hormone beta human chorionic gonadotrophin (βHCG or HCG). The levels of this hormone rise steadily, doubling approximately every 48 hours. Levels rise until around the end of the first trimester. An over-the-counter urine pregnancy test uses a chemical to produce a colour change when HCG is detected in the urine.

Over-the-counter pregnancy tests are extremely accurate and can detect levels of HCG as low as 20 or 50mIU (international units). In the average pregnancy, HCG levels are above 50mIU by the end of the fourth week, or the first day of your missed period. However, if your menstrual cycle tends to fluctuate in length by a few days each month you may have a negative test result if you take it too early as the HCG levels may not yet have risen to the detectable level. If you have a negative pregnancy test and your period does not start, repeat the test after approximately 48 hours; if you are pregnant your HCG levels will have risen and the test may become positive. Even a faint line in the results window is a positive test!

You do not need to go to your GP to confirm a pregnancy as the urine tests used by doctors are the same as those bought over the counter. A blood test can be done to detect the levels of HCG in the bloodstream but the urine tests are accurate enough to confirm pregnancy. Once you have had a positive urine test do make an appointment to see your doctor so that your antenatal care can be put into place. Alternatively, in some places you may be able to book directly with a local midwife, or refer yourself to the local hospital via an online booking service.

Many women want to tell everyone they know as soon as they find out they are pregnant. Other women prefer to wait until the 12-week scan, when the risk of miscarriage has decreased significantly. It is up to you who you tell. Many women probably strike a compromise, perhaps telling close family and friends while waiting to tell others.

'I took a few tests, well quite a few tests! On the day I expected my period I took a test and the line was so faint that I thought I was making myself see something that wasn't there. So the next day I did another one, and again the day after that when finally there was no mistaking it – I was pregnant!' Emily, 31

week 5

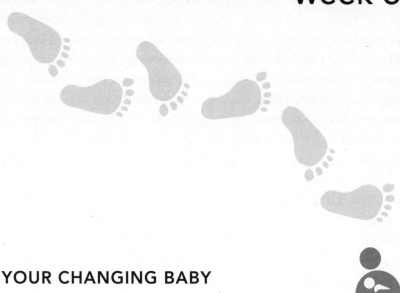

YOUR CHANGING BABY

The blastocyst – the collection of cells that will eventually become your baby – continues to multiply rapidly during the fifth week, and begins to divide into more specialised cells. It is already attached to the wall of your womb. Around half of the cells will eventually form the placenta (which will nourish and support the baby) and surrounding membranes; the other half will form the baby itself. The baby will be connected to the placenta via the umbilical cord, which is also developing. From now until the eighth week, the term embryo is used to describe the baby, after which it is referred to as the foetus. Amniotic fluid begins to form; your baby will float in this fluid throughout your pregnancy (for more information see page 57).

By the end of this week the neural tube develops. This tube is where the brain and spinal cord will form. Your baby's heart also starts to take shape, though as yet it is so small it may not be seen on an ultrasound scan. Soon it will begin to beat, though, at a much faster rate than your own heartbeat. His intestine forms as a hollow tube from where his mouth will be to what is currently his tail, and other major organs such as the kidneys and liver are starting to develop.

A gestational sac containing a yolk sac can be seen on ultrasound scan. The gestational sac is only a few millimetres in diameter and grows about 1mm per day until around the ninth week of pregnancy. The yolk sac provides the growing embryo with its nutritional needs until the placenta is developed and functioning. The size of this sac can be used to calculate the age of the baby. Your baby will have doubled his length from about 2mm to approximately 4mm during this week.

YOUR CHANGING BODY

Although you may have only just found out that you are pregnant, your hormone levels are changing and many adjustments are being made in your body to accommodate your pregnancy. Some women may not notice any symptoms at all, while others may already be feeling tired or nauseous (for more information see Weeks 8 and 9).

You will be producing high levels of the hormone progesterone, which makes the mucus from your cervix very thick. Your cervical mucus normally changes during your menstrual cycle: it becomes very thin before ovulation under the influence of the hormone oestrogen; it then becomes thicker after ovulation under the influence of progesterone. Your levels of progesterone will be higher than normal and so the mucus thickens even more to form a plug in your cervix. This plug helps keep your womb a sterile environment, protecting the uterus and baby from any infections spreading up from the vagina during your pregnancy. It comes out at the start of labour, and is what makes up the 'show'.

The cells which will become your baby and placenta are producing beta human chorionic gonadotrophin (βHCG or HCG), the hormone that turned your pregnancy test positive. The role of HCG is to ensure that you keep producing oestrogen and progesterone from the shell of the egg (corpus luteum) until the placenta is formed and mature enough to take over hormone production. HCG levels rise until about Week 10–12 of pregnancy and then begin to fall. HCG has other roles such as encouraging the thyroid gland to produce more thyroid hormone – thyroxine – to increase your metabolic rate during pregnancy.

'I need to go to the toilet all the time!'

One of the earliest signs of pregnancy is needing to urinate more frequently than previously, and it can feel like you need to go all the time! This is called urinary frequency. The changes that are already happening in your body result in increased blood flow to the kidneys, which receive about 30 per cent more blood than before. The kidneys filter and clean the blood, and have a role in controlling the amount of fluid in your body; the more blood they filter, the more urine may be produced.

Even at this early stage, your growing womb puts pressure on your bladder, which then cannot expand and hold as much urine as previously. So, the combination of producing more urine with less space to hold it makes you need to go to the toilet more often. This symptom often subsides by the end of the first trimester but recurs during the third trimester when there is even less room for your bladder to hold urine.

It is normal to have increased frequency of urine in pregnancy. However, if you need to go even more often than you have come to expect, have lower abdominal pain, or pain or stinging when passing urine, you may have developed a urinary tract infection and should see your doctor.

'I feel like I spend all my time either in the toilet, needing the toilet, wondering where the nearest toilet is, needing the toilet and then going again – all day!'
Anne, 24

PROTECTING YOUR BABY IN THE WOMB

Women are bombarded by often conflicting advice in the press or on the internet about what is healthy and not in pregnancy. It is easy to become frustrated, anxious and overwhelmed. Approximately 4 per cent of babies are born with abnormalities, but of these the majority are due to genetic problems and not related to an infection or toxin. The placenta acts as a barrier to infections and dilutes the effects of many drugs and toxins, though some infections or toxins can pass through. Follow the advice below about staying safe in pregnancy and see your healthcare provider if you have any worries.

You may be concerned that you exposed your baby to a potential hazard before you knew you were pregnant, but try to remember that for the first few weeks of pregnancy the embryo is self-sufficient as it implants and develops. Now is a good time to look at your diet and lifestyle and to try to start being healthy. (For information about a healthy diet and which foods to avoid in pregnancy see Week 7.)

Smoking

We all know that smoking is bad for our health, and that it is addictive and difficult to give up. Smoking during pregnancy affects the normal development of the placenta; your baby may not receive the oxygen and nutrients he needs, resulting in growth restriction. Smoking also increases your risk of a premature delivery so it is best to stop smoking for the health of both you and your baby.

If your partner smokes, inhaling his smoke passively will also have an effect so encourage him to give up as well. Giving up together may be easier as you can support each other. It is never too late to stop smoking, and your doctor will be able to support you and give you smoking cessation advice if you do decide to quit.

Alcohol

The amount of alcohol considered to be safe in pregnancy is currently under debate. In the UK, the National Institute for Clinical Excellence currently recommends that women avoid consuming any alcohol in the first three months of pregnancy. It then advises that very small amounts of alcohol – say one to two units per week or about one glass of wine – are considered safe. Women are advised to avoid getting drunk or binge drinking (drinking over five or six units on any one occasion) during pregnancy.

Large amounts of alcohol, be it through binge drinking or regular consumption, are harmful to the developing foetus and can cause foetal alcohol spectrum disorders or foetal alcohol syndrome, which can result in various problems, both at birth and later in life (see overleaf). In the US women are advised to avoid alcohol altogether during pregnancy. Although it is known that regularly drinking large amounts of alcohol can cause problems with pregnancy, it is not yet clear what is 'safe'. It therefore may be wiser to

'HOW MANY UNITS AM I DRINKING?'

- 1 unit = half a pint of standard strength (5 per cent) beer, lager or cider
- 1 unit = one standard pub measure of spirits
- 1.5 units = one bottle of alcopop
- 1.5–2 units = one glass of standard strength wine (12.5 per cent): 125ml glass = 1.5 units; 175ml glass = 2.1 units
- 9 units = one bottle of standard strength wine

abstain altogether during pregnancy. If you do drink a lot and would like help in cutting down, or if you were not aware of the recommended drink limits and have been drinking more regularly, visit your doctor.

Instead of alcohol, try soft drinks or non-alcoholic cocktails. Try changing your routine to avoid places where you would normally drink, such as the pub. You could ask your partner to also decrease or stop drinking, and support each other during this time. If you have not yet told your friends that you are pregnant and they are

FOETAL ALCOHOL SYNDROME

Foetal alcohol syndrome is thought to affect approximately 1–2 per 100 births. It is a term used to describe a collection of symptoms and signs that occur in babies born to mothers who have regularly drunk large amounts of alcohol (over six units per day) during their pregnancies. The degree of the problem depends on how much alcohol was drunk, whether there was binge drinking and at which point during the pregnancy the alcohol was consumed. The effects on the baby include low birth weight, small head, flat face with a short upturned nose, a thin upper lip, a flat mid face and abnormally slanting eyes. There may be other effects such as heart problems or cleft palate; feeding problems and irritability in these babies is common. In the longer term, these children may have poor growth, learning difficulties and behaviour problems such as hyperactivity.

FOETAL ALCOHOL SPECTRUM DISORDERS

Foetal alcohol spectrum disorders is an umbrella term used to describe a wide range of disorders in babies born to mothers who have regularly drunk over two units per day of alcohol during their pregnancies. Any of the signs of foetal alcohol syndrome may be present to varying degrees, and how severe the condition is depends on how much alcohol has been drunk.

Both foetal alcohol spectrum disorders and foetal alcohol syndrome are lifelong conditions. The children do not grow out of them. They are both preventable by not drinking alcohol during pregnancy.

pressuring you to drink, tell them that you are on a new health drive, or that you are on medication (like antibiotics) and can't drink, and would prefer an orange juice instead!

Medication

Some medicines prescribed by doctors can cause problems. In certain situations a balance has to be struck between the risk to yourself (and the baby) if you stop a medication and the risk to the baby if you continue, for example with anti-epilepsy medication, though do discuss such decisions with your antenatal team. A common example is the use of steroid inhalers for asthma during pregnancy. Asthma sufferers are advised to continue using their inhalers because they have not been shown to cause problems with the baby. In addition, the risks associated with a severe asthma attack, which would affect the amount of oxygen getting to the baby, are greater than any potential risk from the medication. Discuss such decisions with your antenatal team.

Always inform your doctor or pharmacist that you are pregnant before taking any prescribed or over-the-counter remedy so that you can choose one which is known to be safe in pregnancy. For example, use paracetamol as a painkiller instead of ibuprofen, which may cause heart problems in the foetus.

Drugs

Recreational drugs such as heroin and cocaine are illegal. They can cross the placenta and can lead to problems such as premature delivery. Intrauterine growth restriction, where the baby is smaller than expected, is another possible problem; this can result in various complications such as jaundice and difficulty controlling body temperature. Depending on the drug used, your baby may be born addicted to it and suffer withdrawal after birth; this can result in seizures or brain damage.

X-RAYS AND ULTRASOUND SCANS

X-rays are a source of radiation and, in large doses, can be harmful to the developing foetus. Doctors weigh up the risk to the foetus versus the need for the X-ray, and will protect the baby as much as possible using a lead apron to cover your abdomen. Ultrasound scans are considered safe in pregnancy.

If you take recreational drugs, inform your doctor so that your baby can be monitored and helped after birth. Your doctor can also help you to stop. Doctors are bound by laws regarding your confidentiality; they cannot tell anyone, including the police, about your medical history unless they feel you may be putting others at risk. Due to a potential risk to the baby, doctors will tell a social worker that you have taken drugs; not to punish you, but to give you any support that you and your baby may need.

Infections

Most viral coughs and colds will not affect your baby and, as your immune system is lowered slightly during pregnancy, you may get more colds than usual. However, a high fever increases your risk of miscarriage, so use paracetamol and/or tepid sponging or a fan to help bring the fever down. Good food hygiene will help minimise the risk of food poisoning and foods such as raw eggs should be avoided throughout pregnancy to reduce the risk of salmonella infection. Ensure that fish, seafood and chicken are well cooked; wash all fruit and vegetables, and wash your hands after handling raw meat or poultry. When on holiday drink bottled water.

If you have not had chickenpox or been immunised against rubella (German measles) it is advisable to avoid children with these conditions, or children with an undiagnosed rash or fever. Chickenpox increases the risk of early miscarriage and foetal problems such as brain abnormalities. Rubella also increases the risk of miscarriage and foetal abnormalities such as deafness. If you are concerned that you have had contact with an infected child, see your healthcare provider, who may take blood tests to check your immunity and arrange further tests such as ultrasound scans.

Pets

If you have a cat it is important to avoid contact with the litter tray and make sure that your cat is regularly dewormed. Always wash your hands thoroughly after touching a cat. This is to decrease the risk of contracting an infection called toxoplasmosis, which is carried by many cats and can affect the developing baby. Many women are immune but it is sensible to take precautions during pregnancy, so if you do have to handle the litter tray be sure to wear gloves and wash your hands thoroughly afterwards. For other pets, good hygiene is also important so always wash your hands after handling animals.

Beauty treatments

Dyeing your hair
Dyeing or colouring your hair during pregnancy is probably safe, as dyes have been used for many years and there is no evidence that they cause harm. However, as there is also not enough information to say that they are completely safe, many women choose to avoid colouring their hair in the first trimester. Only dye that touches the scalp can be absorbed into your body so having highlights instead of dyeing all your hair may decrease the risk. Vegetable dyes such as henna are considered to be safe.

Waxing
It is safe to continue waxing during pregnancy though you may notice that your skin becomes more sensitive than previously, so you may wish to repeat a patch test. As your pregnancy continues you may find it harder to reach various spots on your body so a salon wax may be more appropriate.

Nail varnish
Nail varnish and having acrylic nails put on are also probably safe in pregnancy but there is not a lot of research on these topics. Any risk is thought to be from solvents used in the treatments, but the doses are probably too small to have any effect.

'WHEN AM I DUE?'
EXPECTED DELIVERY DATES

Your expected delivery date (EDD) is calculated according to your menstrual cycle. The first day of your period is defined as the date of your last menstrual period (LMP). Add 40 weeks to that date and you have your expected delivery date. For example, if your LMP was 14 June, your EDD is 21 March the following year. A pregnancy is considered full term after 37 weeks of pregnancy. The accuracy of your EDD depends on whether or not you have a regular 28-day cycle. If your cycle is longer or shorter the date will be less accurate. Due to this inaccuracy your baby's age and EDD will also be calculated from measurements taken at your 12-week scan (for more information see Week 12).

'HELP! I'M PANICKING'

At this stage in pregnancy many women find themselves preoccupied with countless questions, concerns and fears. The initial reaction to being pregnant, be it joy and delight or shock, may be replaced with worries: 'Will my baby be okay?' 'Will I have a miscarriage?' Before you knew you were pregnant you may have got very drunk, eaten lots of Brie or been in contact with someone with an infectious disease, and now you are worried that it will affect the baby. You may also be anxious about telling people, how you will manage at work and so on. These and countless other fears may go round and round in your thoughts and can become distressing.

The first thing to do is stop and take a deep breath. It is perfectly okay, and in fact normal, to feel overwhelmed or scared. A huge thing is happening to your body and to your life, and thinking about it is the natural way to start to deal with the changes that are occurring. Your worries may be influenced by things that happened to women in your family or to your friends, or in your own past. Remember that in the majority of cases pregnancy is uneventful and produces a healthy bouncing baby! Don't bottle everything up inside: talk about your concerns to your partner, your friends or family if you have told them you are pregnant, or to your doctor. Sometimes even just writing things down can help. Once you start talking you will probably find that most women have felt the same way at some point during pregnancy or motherhood, and although this may not negate your fears it can help you manage your concerns.

'I have rational thoughts and then crazy lady thoughts. For example, one minute I am literally jumping with joy and the next am in a heap on the floor wondering whether everything will turn out okay. Rational head says that I am healthy, and there is no reason to worry; crazy head then screams something else! I am hoping that at some point rational head will win!' Patricia, 32

week 6

YOUR CHANGING BABY

Your baby's face has started to develop. Currently he has a very large head with tiny openings where his mouth and nostrils will be, and what look like dark patches which will turn into his eyes. He has small folds on either side of his head that will become his ears. Limb buds are present which will develop into arms and legs with paddle-shaped hands, and he even has the beginnings of what will become his fingers and toes.

The first blood vessels and blood cells are forming, and blood begins to flow through these vessels. His heart now starts to flutter and can be seen on an ultrasound scan. His spinal cord and spine are developing more quickly than the rest of his body at the moment so it looks like he has a little tail, like a tadpole, but the rest of him will soon catch up.

Your baby is floating in a sac filled with all the nutrients he needs until the placenta is fully formed and functioning in a few weeks' time. This sac is only about 14mm (0.5 inch) wide, and the embryo itself is still less than a centimetre long (on average 4–7mm), about the length of a grain of rice, yet he is developing very rapidly. An ultrasound scan at this stage would detect the gestational sac, within which the foetal pole, which will become your baby, would be visible.

YOUR CHANGING BODY

Your uterus is already beginning to get bigger. This difference may be felt if your doctor were to examine you internally. There is a long way to go – your womb will increase up to a thousand times its normal size during pregnancy. The volume of blood in your body starts to increase. Your heart is pumping harder and faster than before to get the blood – and the oxygen and glucose carried in your blood – to your organs and the baby. By the time the baby comes you will have about 1.5 times the amount of blood in your body than before you were pregnant, an increase from approximately 5 litres to 7.5 litres (about 8¾–13 pints). You will currently be producing more plasma, the liquid part of your blood, and later will also produce more red blood cells. The supply of blood to your uterus will have doubled already and will continue to increase up to the end of pregnancy. Blood supply to other organs such as your breasts, kidneys and skin also increases. You cannot feel this change happening but you may have noticed that the skin of your vagina and vulva has become darker, almost purple in colour, which is a sign of this increased blood flow.

Breast changes and tenderness

The increasing levels of hormones such as progesterone affect not only your womb but your breasts too, which tend to get bigger during the first trimester. Most women find that they increase a couple of cup sizes in a very short space of time but then don't have any changes for a few months, before growing again towards the end of pregnancy. Others may find that their breasts grow more gradually. Wearing a soft bra at night can be helpful, especially if your breasts are large, to provide support.

As your breasts get bigger you may notice that you develop more obvious veins across them, reflecting the increased blood supply to them. Your breasts may also feel tender or firmer, similar to what you might have felt previously when your period was due. In fact, your breasts may become so tender that sleeping on your front is uncomfortable. Again, wearing a bra at night can help, and some people find an aloe vera or camomile cream soothing. Some women notice that their breasts become lumpy, though if you do notice a new lump visit your GP to have it checked.

Your nipples can also change. You may develop little bumps around the areola (the coloured skin around the nipple) that can look like goose bumps. Don't worry – these are normal sweat glands (Montgomery's tubercles) which increase in size. They have a role in lubricating your nipples, preventing them from drying out, and may also help to prevent infection. They generally shrink back down and disappear after pregnancy and breastfeeding.

Bras for pregnancy

A good bra can make you feel good about yourself, enhancing your assets as well as supporting them. A well-fitting bra is a must for all women to support the weight of the breasts, but it becomes even more important during pregnancy. Your breasts are increasing in size and becoming heavy; without the support of a good bra you may develop chest or back pain. Supporting your breasts now may also help prevent them sagging later.

'I was very worried about the fact that I was pregnant with my first child at the age of 43, although I felt prepared both psychologically and financially, and I was really ready for a baby. I wanted to know what effects my age might have on my pregnancy as I knew that older women have an increased risk of having children with Down's syndrome. My doctor was very reassuring and told me about all the tests we could have. It was good to be able to express my concerns.' Jane, 44

Don't put off buying bras thinking that you will only need new ones in a few weeks' time. That may be the case, but most women find that their breasts get bigger rapidly at the beginning of their pregnancy before the speed of growth slows down. A good shop assistant will also be able to help you pick a bra that should last you even if your breasts do change a little. Lots of consumer research has shown that many women are wearing the wrong size bra, so do get fitted by a bra fitter and tell her that you are pregnant. You should have your bust measured every four weeks during pregnancy to ensure that you are still wearing correctly fitting bras.

A pregnancy or maternity bra is very supportive, with wide straps and a wide band under the cup to support and spread the weight of the breasts. You can find many pretty or sexy maternity bras. Sports bras are similar, and many women choose to wear them during pregnancy. Underwired bras are not recommended in pregnancy as the bigger you get, the more the wire may dig into the breast; this is not only uncomfortable but may damage the breast tissue itself. If you do still decide to wear an underwired bra, it is important that it fits properly.

REGISTERING WITH YOUR DOCTOR

Your first antenatal appointment can be with your GP or you may be able to book directly with a local midwife. You can do this as soon as you find out that you are pregnant, or you may prefer to wait a couple of weeks, but this appointment should be relatively early in the first trimester as the aim is that you will be able to have a booking appointment before 12 weeks (see Week 11). At that appointment your doctor will ask you various questions about your health and any previous pregnancies. This is called your medical history, and from this your doctor will be able to make decisions (with you) about the care that is most appropriate for you during your pregnancy.

If you have a known medical condition or had a problem in a previous pregnancy, your doctor will be able to arrange appropriate care or any tests that may be required. If you are taking medication, this will be discussed with you; certain medications may be changed or even stopped (for more information about medications in pregnancy see page 19). Always tell any doctors or pharmacists that you are pregnant so appropriate medication can be prescribed. Certain conditions may improve during pregnancy, while others may flare up after delivery.

At your booking appointment you will also be given some lifestyle advice, such as on alcohol intake and the importance of taking folic acid supplements. If you smoke, this is a good opportunity to discuss quitting, and to find out how your doctor can help. Your doctor may also discuss the structure of antenatal care (see Week 9), screening tests and scans. Your blood pressure will be taken at this appointment.

You may be asked to sign a form declaring that you are pregnant. Your doctor also signs this form and sends it to the relevant agency so that you will receive a maternity exemption card in the post. If you show this card at any pharmacy, you will not be charged the prescription fee. You are entitled to free prescriptions throughout your pregnancy and for one year after your expected delivery date.

This first visit, as with all your antenatal appointments, is an opportunity for you to discuss any concerns or questions you may have, no matter how simple you feel they are. Do ask, as many women find that there are reassuring answers to their questions, or benefit from simply discussing their concerns.

Antenatal care options

After taking your history your doctor or midwife will discuss with you what kind of antenatal care you would like. The purpose of antenatal care is to monitor your pregnancy to ensure that you and your baby stay healthy. There are various options, involving obstetricians, GPs and midwives, and what is available may differ between areas.

- Complete hospital-based or consultant-led care: you are looked after by, and have all your antenatal appointments with, an obstetrician (specialist in the care of pregnant women) in the hospital.

- Shared care: you attend hospital once or twice and deliver your baby there but the rest of your antenatal appointments are with your GP or midwives outside the hospital in your doctor's surgery (anything outside the hospital is often referred to as 'in the community'). In this way your care is 'shared' between the hospital and the community.
- GP-led care: you see your GP for all your routine appointments. Your delivery may be in the hospital or at home.
- Midwifery-led care: you are looked after by a team of midwives, generally in the community, though still under the auspices of a hospital. You will only see a doctor if there is a complication. You can have your baby in the hospital. In some midwifery schemes you will be looked after during labour by one of the midwives who saw you during your pregnancy, as in a Domino scheme (see below); in others you may be looked after by one set of midwives during your pregnancy and another during labour.
- Domino scheme: this is available in some, but not all, hospitals. You are looked after by a team of midwives in the community, and one of these midwives will visit you at home when you are in labour. They will then go to the hospital with you and look after you throughout your labour, unless complications arise, in which case your care will be transferred to the midwives and doctors in the hospital.
- Independent midwives: these are fully trained, qualified midwives who do not work in the NHS. Instead, you pay for their services and receive care from the same midwife antenatally, during your labour and postnatally, enabling good continuity of care. You could also pay for private care by an obstetrician or a combination of private obstetrician and midwife.

Every pregnancy is different, so a woman's choice of antenatal care is always an individual one. She may require different types of care for different pregnancies. If you have a known medical condition or have had a previous condition during pregnancy, it may be recommended that you are cared for by the hospital obstetricians.

However, the majority of pregnancies are healthy and therefore considered low-risk so shared care, GP- or midwifery-led care in the community is appropriate. Remember, if the situation changes your midwife can always refer you to a doctor. Discuss the options with your GP so together you can decide the best antenatal care for your pregnancy (for more information see 'Where should I have my baby?', page 60).

FOR FATHERS

For the man it can feel like all the focus in pregnancy is on the woman and how she is feeling, both physically and emotionally. However, just as she will have concerns, questions and anxieties about the pregnancy, so may you; after all, both your lives are changing dramatically. Common anxieties among men include how the baby will affect their relationship or their finances, as perhaps they will become the sole breadwinner for a while. You may find it difficult to watch your partner being unwell, or in pain during labour.

It can be difficult for men to stay involved during the pregnancy. Although they can see the changes happening to their partner's body, men do not experience them in the same way. So try to get involved. Go to antenatal appointments and actively take part in

'So, we're pregnant, except really she's pregnant not me, though we are having a baby. It is weird – my sperm, her egg, half her, half me – but now there's all this stuff going on in her body but as yet nothing has changed for me. It might be silly but I'm already putting my hand on her tummy – that's my baby in there!' Daniel, 29

them: ask questions; get involved in discussions; read any information given. Go with your partner to the scans so you can see your baby. Take the time to talk and listen to each other. Remember, having a baby is happening to both of you!

week 7

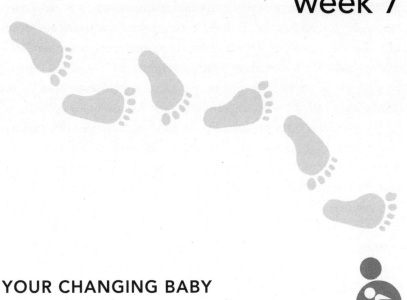

YOUR CHANGING BABY

Your baby is just beginning to straighten up from his curled-over comma shape, though he still looks like a tadpole with a long back in relation to the length of his limbs. The red blood cells that carry oxygen round the body start to be produced by the baby's liver, taking over from the yolk sac. When your baby's bones are formed, the bone marrow will be the producer of blood cells.

Your baby's skin is translucent and very thin; his face continues to develop; his ears, palate and nose are forming, along with the lenses in his eyes. The paddle-shaped hands and feet are changing, with the fingers and toes becoming more defined and webbed. He is beginning to move around; the movements are jerky and can be seen on an ultrasound scan by this point. Your baby is approximately a centimetre in length (less than half an inch).

YOUR CHANGING BODY

Although your womb is getting bigger it is still small and contained within the bones of your pelvis. It rises out of the pelvis into the abdomen at about the end of the first trimester when it can be felt through your abdomen. In order for enough oxygen and nutrients to reach your growing womb and breasts, and to supply your developing baby, the speed of your metabolism increases during pregnancy by up to 25 per cent. Your heart also has to pump a lot harder to get the increased amount of blood round your body.

You will be producing lots of the hormone oestrogen during your pregnancy. At this early stage it is still being produced by the corpus luteum (shell of the egg), but it will mainly be produced by the placenta once it is formed and functioning. Your baby is also involved in the production of oestrogen, irrespective of its sex. Oestrogen has many roles and effects; it is involved in the growth of your breasts and womb, and helps increase the blood supply to your body. It also affects your skin and hair, contributing to the rosy cheeks and shiny hair traditionally associated with the 'glow of pregnancy'. It also has a role in softening components of your connective tissue to allow it to become more flexible to accommodate your growing baby and womb.

BLEEDING IN EARLY PREGNANCY

Bleeding during the first trimester of pregnancy is extremely common, affecting up to one in three pregnant women. It does not always mean that you are having a miscarriage. A miscarriage is the loss of an embryo or foetus within the first 24 weeks of pregnancy, though it is more likely to occur in the very early stages of pregnancy, most often in the first few weeks (see below). The amount of blood can vary from a few dots or spots to copious amounts of blood with lots of clots; this blood is not coming from the baby but from you or the lining of your womb. Bleeding can be associated with pain or cramping in the lower abdomen.

Any bleeding in pregnancy should be investigated by a doctor. You will be examined vaginally and generally offered an early ultrasound. Scans carried out early in the first trimester are usually performed transvaginally, that is with a small probe in the vagina, as the embryo is too small to be seen through the abdomen. For many women, the bleeding resolves and there are no effects to the foetus. Doctors may not be able to say why some bleeding has occurred, though for other women it may have a more obvious cause, such as an infection.

Miscarriage

The risk of miscarriage decreases the further along in your pregnancy you are. The majority of miscarriages occur very early on in pregnancy, often even before you know you are pregnant. By the end of the first trimester the risk of miscarriage is as low as 1 per cent, so 99 in every 100 pregnancies that reach 12 weeks will continue. Although bleeding is extremely frightening and should be investigated (see above), it does not mean a miscarriage is inevitable; the embryo may still be fine.

Many women worry that they did something to cause a miscarriage, but do try to remember that a miscarriage is no one's fault; it just happens. Miscarriage can be hugely upsetting for both partners and you will need time to recover, physically and emotionally. Counselling and miscarriage support groups are available if you feel you would find them helpful. Your doctor should be able to guide you further.

'I remember thinking that I would never stay pregnant, that there must be something wrong with me. When I did get pregnant the doctors and midwives were great, arranging an extra early scan because I was so worried, but as soon as I got to 12 weeks I relaxed. Fast forward two years and I've got a toddler pottering around and another one on the way!' April, 39

DIET IN PREGNANCY

A healthy diet in pregnancy is basically the same as a healthy diet outside pregnancy – balanced and varied in carbohydrates, proteins, fats, vitamins and minerals. Your calorie needs barely increase in the first trimester. By the third trimester you will need only approximately 200–300 calories per day more than normal, which is only an extra two slices of bread! In fact, breastfeeding requires more energy from calories in food than pregnancy does, about an extra 500 calories per day.

Pregnancy is a good time to look at your diet to see if you can improve what you are eating. However, remember that it is very common for women in the first trimester to feel nauseous and not eat very much, or to eat strange and restrictive combinations of food. Try not to worry about this. As long as you are drinking enough fluids your baby will be getting the nutrients he needs from your body.

Carbohydrates

These are broken down in the body to form energy. Simple carbohydrates such as sweets or biscuits are easily broken down to sugars, so they give a short burst of energy that is quickly used up. Complex carbohydrates such as potatoes, porridge or pulses take longer to be broken down and so give a slow, steady supply of energy. Wholegrain, wholemeal or brown carbohydrates are broken down more slowly than 'white' versions. You should aim for four to six servings of complex carbohydrates per day, such as brown bread, pasta or rice.

Protein

Protein is used to create the organs, bones and tissues of your and your baby's body. In pregnancy, you need about a fifth more protein than previously, even from the first trimester. Protein is found in meat, poultry, fish, dairy, pulses and nuts. Aim to eat two to three servings of protein per day. A serving is about 85 grams (3 ounces), or a piece of meat, poultry or fish approximately the size of a deck of playing cards or the palm of your hand. Try to eat at least two portions of fish per week, including at least one portion of oily fish. Most fish is safe but some should be avoided (for more information see 'What shouldn't I eat?', overleaf).

Fats

Many women think that they should avoid fats in their diet entirely. Fats, however, are an essential part of your diet, especially when you are pregnant. Among other things, fats are needed to dissolve certain vitamins in the body. Healthy fats are unsaturated and include those found in nuts and vegetable oils; unhealthy fats are saturated and are found in fried and processed foods.

Dairy

It is important to eat dairy produce that contains calcium and vitamins; semi-skimmed milk can be used instead of full-fat milk as it contains approximately the same amount of calcium.

Fruit and vegetables

You should aim to eat at least five portions of fruit and vegetables per day (fruit juice counts as only one portion, no matter how much you drink). Aim to eat varied and colourful fruit and vegetables to ensure you are getting a wide range of vitamins and minerals (for more information see Week 19).

Fluids

Fluids are just as important as the food you eat. You need to drink 2 litres per day. The best liquid to drink is water but you can vary it with some fruit juice or milk.

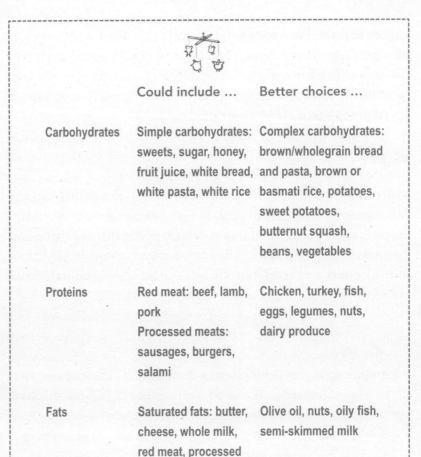

	Could include ...	Better choices ...
Carbohydrates	Simple carbohydrates: sweets, sugar, honey, fruit juice, white bread, white pasta, white rice	Complex carbohydrates: brown/wholegrain bread and pasta, brown or basmati rice, potatoes, sweet potatoes, butternut squash, beans, vegetables
Proteins	Red meat: beef, lamb, pork Processed meats: sausages, burgers, salami	Chicken, turkey, fish, eggs, legumes, nuts, dairy produce
Fats	Saturated fats: butter, cheese, whole milk, red meat, processed meats	Olive oil, nuts, oily fish, semi-skimmed milk

As you can see, some foods contain more than one element, such as protein as well as fat. So, although dairy produce such as cheese or yoghurt may contain saturated fats, it is also a good source of protein (and calcium) and still fine to eat – everything in moderation!

'What shouldn't I eat?'

There is a lot of information in the press about what women should and shouldn't eat during pregnancy. This can be confusing and even conflicting. In fact, only a few foods should be actively avoided during pregnancy – foods that can make you or your baby unwell. (For more information about safety in pregnancy, see Week 5.)

- **Liver or liver products** contain very high levels of vitamin A which can be toxic to the developing foetus.
- **Raw or undercooked eggs** carry a risk of salmonella food poisoning. Choose eggs that have been cooked so that both the white and the yolk are firm. This often means avoiding certain desserts made with raw eggs, such as mousses, home-made mayonnaise or ice creams. Bought mayonnaise and ice cream are generally made with pasteurised eggs and so are considered safe. If you are unsure, check the label or ask!
- **Pâtés and soft unpasteurised cheeses** such as Brie or Camembert, and **blue cheeses** such as Stilton and Gorgonzola, carry a risk of listeria infection, which can be harmful to the baby. Safe cheeses include hard cheeses, mozzarella, feta cheese, goat's cheese without a white rind, cottage cheese, ricotta, mascarpone, cream cheeses, crème fraîche, fromage frais and processed cheeses such as Dairylea.
- **Undercooked or raw meat, poultry and fish** should be avoided to decrease the risk of food poisoning. Make sure you wash your hands after handling raw meat. Sushi bought at a supermarket, which has been pasteurised or flash frozen, can be eaten. It is not possible to know how the fish in a restaurant has been treated, so it is probably best avoided.
- **Fish that are high in mercury** should be avoided – these are shark, marlin and swordfish. Tuna does contain mercury, though at lower levels, so you can eat two tuna steaks (weighing about 170g each raw) or four medium cans of tuna (drained weight 140g in each can) per week. Don't forget to include the tuna in any bought sandwiches. Avoid having more than two portions of oily fish a week, including trout, sardines and fresh (but not canned) tuna.
- **Raw shellfish** should also be avoided as it can cause food poisoning.

CAFFEINE

It is recommended that pregnant women limit their intake of caffeine as high levels have been associated with low birth weight babies and miscarriage. Caffeine acts as a diuretic, making you urinate more and drink more. It also interferes with and blocks the absorption of some vitamins and minerals from your diet, such as iron and vitamin C.

The Food Standards Agency recommends that you consume no more than 200mg of caffeine per day during pregnancy. Caffeine is found in tea, coffee, cola and chocolate and can be added to energy drinks. The average mug of coffee contains 100mg of caffeine, a mug of tea 75mg, a 50g bar of dark chocolate 50mg, a 50g bar of milk chocolate 25mg and a can of cola about 40mg. So you can have one cup of coffee and two chocolate bars! The amount of caffeine in a large mug of coffee from a coffee shop may be significantly more than the averages mentioned above. Some herbal teas, such as green tea, also contain caffeine so always check the label.

Alcohol

It is recommended that you cut out all alcohol for the first three months of pregnancy, after which one or two units (about one glass of wine) per week is currently considered to be safe (for more information see Week 5).

What about nuts?

If you are allergic to nuts you should avoid them at any time, not just during pregnancy! It is not known whether eating or avoiding nuts changes the risk of your baby developing a nut allergy. If your partner or other children have severe nut allergies you may wish to avoid nuts while you are pregnant. Research is being carried out into this topic so the recommendations may change. Contact your doctor for the latest advice.

> 'Everyone tells me different things – eat this, don't eat this, if you eat that you're a bad mother – so instead of listening to lots of different opinions I bought one book and stuck to it. Blue cheese was out but apart from that I didn't need to change my diet much at all. In fact, I was eating the healthiest I had done in ages.'
> Stacey, 34

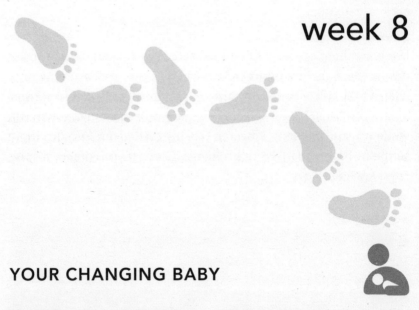

week 8

YOUR CHANGING BABY

The embryo is now called a foetus and is beginning to look more like a newborn as his embryonic 'tail' disappears. His spinal column is forming and his bones are starting to develop; his arms and legs have got longer with the site of knee, elbow, wrist and ankle defined. His head is still very large and bent forward with his chin attached to his chest; inside his head his brain develops further, separating into two hemispheres. He is moving, though you won't feel the movements for many weeks yet as he is still very small and can't create big enough ripples in the amniotic fluid for you to feel them.

The intestines continue to develop and the stomach becomes more defined. Your baby's face develops further; the eyelids begin to develop though his eyes are still fused shut. He has all his teeth buds, though he won't be teething until he is at least a few months old. He is about 1.5 centimetres (0.6 inch) long and, although all his major organs are forming, he weighs approximately 1 gram (0.04 ounces).

YOUR CHANGING BODY

Your uterus is continuing to grow and needs an increased blood supply to provide it with its oxygen and glucose requirements.

Normally, when you are not pregnant, your womb does not need a very big blood supply, but by the end of the first trimester it takes about one quarter of the blood pumped out with each heartbeat. Your heart rate increases slightly and your heart pumps out more blood with each beat. The hormone progesterone is involved in this process by relaxing the tissue in the walls of the heart so it can fill with more blood and therefore pump more out with each heartbeat.

Progesterone has many other roles. It acts to relax your blood vessels, so that they can cope with the increased blood flow around your body without increasing your blood pressure. This works so well that your blood pressure generally falls during pregnancy. Progesterone relaxes your digestive system, which can cause constipation. It also stops your womb from contracting until it is time for labour, and has a role in helping to loosen connective tissue in ligaments and tendons so that your body can cope with your growing womb. Progesterone affects your breasts, preparing them for milk production.

Another pregnancy hormone is human placental lactogen (HPL), which is produced by the placenta. HPL affects your blood sugar levels and insulin production (the hormone which controls your blood sugar levels) to divert stores of glucose and nutrients to your baby. HPL also affects your breast development during pregnancy and milk production after the baby is born. Although you may notice changes in your breasts you will not be aware of the other effects that HPL has on your body.

'WHY DO I FEEL SO SICK?'

The term 'morning sickness' is misleading: most women are not actually sick but feel nauseous, and it can occur at any time during the day, not just in the morning. It is sometimes referred to simply as 'nausea and vomiting in pregnancy'. Symptoms range from mild nausea to vomiting on multiple occasions during the day. Even if you are managing to eat and drink only small amounts, your baby will still be getting its requirements from your body. Up to 80 per cent of women experience some nausea during the first trimester. Not having nausea doesn't mean there is anything wrong – you are just one of the lucky one in five women who don't have these unpleasant symptoms.

There are various theories as to why nausea and vomiting occur during pregnancy. It may be related to the high levels of the hormone human chorionic gonadotrophin (HCG) in the first trimester. HCG levels begin to fall at the end of the first trimester, which correlates with the time most women begin to feel better (around 12–14 weeks). The hormone progesterone may also be involved as it relaxes the muscles of your digestive system; food and stomach acids pass through your stomach more slowly than normal, which may contribute to the feelings of nausea. Symptoms may also be related to low blood sugar levels, as they are traditionally worse in the morning or at a time when you are hungry and your blood sugars are low.

In a rare condition affecting about 1 per cent of women, the vomiting is so severe and prolonged that they cannot keep any fluids down and become dehydrated. This is called hyperemesis gravidarum and needs hospital admission and treatment with intravenous fluids and antiemetic (anti-sickness) medication. If you are concerned that you are unable to drink anything without vomiting, your lips and mouth are becoming dry and your urine is becoming very concentrated (dark in colour and strong smelling) or you are only passing very small amounts of urine infrequently, then visit your doctor.

'I know that it must be harder for her, being the one who feels sick most of the day, but it is also hard for me watching her feel unwell or actually being sick. I feel like it is my fault, like I am making her feel this way. She appears to be fine with it, just accepts it as part of pregnancy and something that will pass, but I find it hard to watch her.' Thomas, 32

Remedies for nausea and vomiting

There are various remedies for nausea and vomiting during pregnancy, though unfortunately there is no magic cure-all. Try different things to see what helps you. If all else fails and you are finding the nausea and/or vomiting difficult to manage, visit your doctor who will be able to prescribe you an anti-sickness medication that is safe in pregnancy.

- Ginger is a traditional remedy for nausea. Try ginger tea or ginger biscuits.
- Peppermint is another traditional remedy. Take it as peppermint tea or sweets, or even put some peppermint oil on a tissue and smell it when you feel nauseous.
- Avoid fatty or greasy foods as they often worsen nausea.
- Try to eat little and often. You may not be able to manage a big meal so eat small snacks regularly. Make sure you have something in your handbag in case you are out and get hungry.
- Try plain foods such as toast, crackers or cereals.
- If you feel worse in the morning it may be related to low blood sugar levels so try eating something like a plain biscuit or cracker before you get out of bed.
- Some women find complementary therapies such as acupuncture or acupressure bands useful for nausea.

Although you may feel awful your baby will be getting everything he needs, even if you are not eating very much. It is important to try and drink so sip water regularly throughout the day.

EXERCISE IN PREGNANCY

We all should exercise. Exercise can be continued, and is in fact encouraged, during pregnancy. You may have to make some modifications to how you exercise as you get bigger (for more information see Weeks 13 and 30). There is a misconception that exercise can cause miscarriage or harm your baby's development, but unless your doctors have specifically told you otherwise, exercise is safe in pregnancy. You may be advised not to exercise if you have, for instance, certain heart conditions or a low-lying placenta (see Week 34), if you are at risk of or have previously had a premature labour, or if your waters have broken.

Blood flow to the uterus actually increases during exercise so your baby continues to get enough of the nutrients and oxygen he needs. Professional endurance athletes may have small babies but the average woman does not do the same amount of exercise as a professional athlete or marathon runner! Remember, the Western lifestyle involves far less exercise than it used to; working women in the developing world are generally far more active, and they have been having babies for years! Avoid contact sports such as boxing, or dangerous sports such as rock climbing. Sports that require balance, such as cycling or horse riding, will become more difficult as you develop a bump and so should also be avoided. Try swimming or walking instead.

Exercise has many benefits: it increases your stamina and (although it sounds contradictory) can actually make you feel more energetic. The fitter you are, the better able your body will be to cope with the demands of pregnancy and labour, meaning you will be less short of breath after climbing stairs when you have a big bump! Working out keeps you strong, supple and flexible and can help with, among many other symptoms, backache and constipation. It will also make it easier for you to get back into shape once the baby has arrived.

Exercise releases endorphins in the body, helping you feel uplifted and relaxed. Your baby also receives this feel-good hormone, making him feel relaxed too. Babies enjoy being rocked, and in the womb they may find the effects of you exercising enjoyable. Finally, you may make new friends at antenatal exercise groups, or spend fun time with your partner at the same time as keeping him in shape!

Before exercising, make sure you have eaten properly that day (though not just before exercising or you may feel unwell). Keep a bottle of water handy. Wear layers so that you can peel off some clothing as you get warmer to prevent yourself from overheating. As your pregnancy progresses you may need to buy new trainers if your feet have swollen. As always, make sure that you warm up and cool down properly with stretches.

If you were working out regularly before pregnancy, such as going for a weekly run or swim, then you should be able to continue as before. You can carry on training with weights, though be sure that you are using the correct technique to prevent injury. You may want to decrease the weights slightly and increase your repetitions to avoid potential harm. Running is hard on the joints, which loosen in pregnancy, so you may be more prone to injury, though running on a track or grass is easier on the joints than running on the road. As your pregnancy continues and your bump gets bigger you may find yourself naturally slowing down but don't worry – even a fast walk counts as exercise! As always, try to ensure that you are using the correct technique for each exercise and don't push yourself too hard.

If you are a beginner to exercise you can start during pregnancy. Aim to exercise at least three times per week, though do allow yourself recovery time in between sessions. When you are working out you should be slightly short of breath but still be able to talk comfortably. Sessions should be approximately 30 minutes long, though you may need to build up to this. It is fine to split your exercise into two or three shorter sessions throughout the day. Every form of activity counts, from walking, climbing the stairs and dancing to housework! Once your bump gets bigger you should avoid lying flat on your back to do exercises, as the weight of your bump may impair the passage of blood up to your heart, decreasing the amount of blood going to the placenta and, in turn, the oxygen and glucose to your baby.

Most importantly, listen to your body and slow down when it tells you to. Exercise has many health benefits and can make you feel fantastic, but if you are feeling tired or nauseous don't overexert yourself. Instead, pace yourself. If you feel up to exercising as before then continue, but if you want to take a break, it is also fine. You will know what is best for you.

'I'M GOING TO BE A SINGLE MUM'

Pregnancy books and magazines are full of images of happy couples but not every pregnant woman is in a traditional relationship. If you are going to be a single mother, for example, you may be intimidated by the thought of going to antenatal classes alone. You could ask a close friend or family member to be your birth partner. Alternatively, you could go to a class designed for single parents, if one is available in your area. Similarly, if you are in a same-sex relationship, you might find it helpful to attend a class or support group for women in your situation. Remember, though, that whatever your circumstances, other women in any antenatal class will share many of your questions and concerns about having a baby. Try to build up a group of people who will support you, perhaps family, friends or people in a similar position to you so you can help each other when needed.

'I was so glad that I went to a single-parenting group. Meeting other women and men in my position has been invaluable in helping me feel supported, and knowing that other people have the same worries as I do really helps put them into perspective.' Toni, 28

week 9

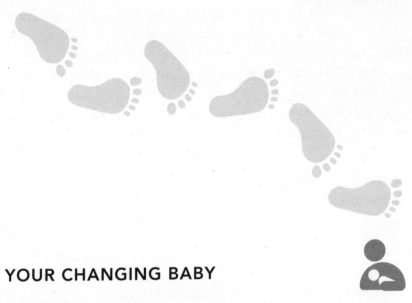

YOUR CHANGING BABY

Although your baby's sex cannot yet be seen on an ultrasound scan, its genitals are beginning to form. Up until the ninth week of pregnancy, genitals are the same for both boy and girl babies; after this point they start to change into the appearance of a boy or a girl.

Your baby's fingers and toes are becoming more defined, as are his facial features; he has a tip to his nose and an upper lip. His tongue is also beginning to develop. His eyes are still shut and will remain so until about Week 26–28 of pregnancy. The baby's head appears very large as his brain is growing very quickly; it is possible to measure his brainwaves at this stage, showing brain activity. He continues to move around and cartilage is beginning to develop. He is about 2.5 centimetres (1 inch) in length and has doubled in weight to about 2 grams (0.07 ounces).

YOUR CHANGING BODY

By this stage in your pregnancy you may have noticed that you have more discharge from your vagina than before you were pregnant. The amount of vaginal discharge you have normally varies with your menstrual cycle. During pregnancy it is thin and watery, generally clear or whitish in colour, without an offensive smell. Vaginal discharge increases due to the effect of your hormones. It is a mixture of secretions and cells from your vagina. See your GP if your discharge becomes yellow or green, offensive in smell or associated with soreness or itching as you may have an infection that needs treating (for more information see Week 30).

'I'm only nine weeks pregnant so why am I so exhausted?'

Feelings of fatigue or even exhaustion are extremely common in early pregnancy. Women are often concerned about their feelings of tiredness as fatigue is associated with being unwell; however, it is not a cause for worry and is natural during pregnancy.

It is not clear why women often feel so tired during the first trimester; it may be related to the many physiological changes that are happening to your body and your developing baby and/or the high levels of hormones in your body. Tiredness can occur at any time but generally worsens as the day goes on. These feelings of utter exhaustion often peak in the first 10 weeks of pregnancy and then tend to improve. By the second trimester you will probably be feeling back to your normal self. In fact, you may even have more energy than normal, though the tiredness does tend to return in late pregnancy.

The combination of feeling nauseous or vomiting and feeling worn out with fatigue can make the first trimester trying for some women. Try to listen to your body. Take naps and have lie-ins if and when you can. Hopefully you will soon be feeling more energetic.

Eating in the first trimester

Eating in the first trimester can be a minefield. You know that you are supposed to eat a varied and healthy diet but you may be feeling nauseous and unable to face many foods. Alternatively, you may have

ENERGY BOOSTERS

If you are suffering from fatigue you might like to consider some energy-boosting snacks to help you get through the day. Avoid sugary snacks such as sweets or chocolate as these will give you a quick burst of energy but, as your blood sugar levels then plummet, you may feel worse than before. Such snacks may also make you put on weight. Try energy-filled snacks such as a banana, a fruit smoothie, a couple of pieces of wholegrain toast, some granola or a handful of nuts and raisins. Easily portable snacks to carry in your handbag are pieces of fruit, bags of nuts, crackers or cereal bars. Avoid energy drinks as these contain extremely high amounts of caffeine (see Week 7).

cravings for a very restricted or even bizarre selection of foods. Even if you are not eating very much your baby will still be getting everything he needs from your body, and as long as you are managing to eat the occasional food and are drinking enough you should be all right, no matter how sick you feel.

During the first trimester you do not need any extra calories per day so try to eat as normal. Many women do not put on any weight, or put on very little weight, during the first trimester; some women even lose weight due to their nausea and vomiting. If you are managing to eat normally then try and stick to a healthy diet. (For more information about nausea and vomiting in pregnancy see Week 8.)

'My daily diet consists of a combination of dry crackers, Hula Hoops and Polos, all washed down by water that is icy cold, even though I know this isn't really healthy. Sometimes I also fancy drinking milk, something I never would have done before. I've gone off things I used to enjoy – that first cup of coffee in the morning or a rich fudgy chocolate cake. Just a cracker or a Hula Hoop sandwich for me!' Catherine, 28

'My mood swings are like PMT but worse. What is happening?'

You might find that you are more emotional or irritable than normal, have mood swings or just feel emotionally fragile. Pregnancy is a time of great change, whether or not you have had children previously. This emotional upheaval, combined with feelings of tiredness, nausea and your rapidly changing hormone levels, means that you may feel your emotions are out of control.

You might find yourself snapping at your partner, easily irritated or crying much more often than usual. It can be difficult for your partner to cope with your changes in mood; indeed, you may find yourself lashing out or crying at something he says that previously you would have laughed at. Try to communicate with him. Remember that these mood swings are not permanent. Explain to him as much as you can about how you are feeling.

SEX IN THE FIRST TRIMESTER

Before discussing anything else about sex, it is
important to say that sex is safe in pregnancy.
Your body will change and your libido may increase
or decrease or go completely crazy. Rest assured,
however, that unless your doctor specifically tells
you to avoid sex (and there are very few situations
where this is the case, such as a low-lying placenta)
it is safe for you to carry on. Not only does sex
release endorphins to make you feel good, it is
physical exercise and a method of keeping
connected to your partner.

Feelings of exhaustion and nausea may mean that
your sex drive decreases during the first trimester.
If you are feeling unwell you may simply not be in
the mood to have sex. If this is the case then explain
your feelings to your partner who will hopefully
understand. You can remain physically close without
having sexual intercourse; plenty of cuddles, massage
and foreplay can keep you physically connected. As
you begin to feel better during the second trimester,
your libido will hopefully return to normal. In fact,
many women report that sex actually improves
during this stage of their pregnancy.

'Between the nausea and the tiredness my sex drive fell to absolute zero, and all I really wanted was a cuddle and then to go to sleep. But when I began to feel better my libido returned to normal, or even better than before!' Natalie, 26

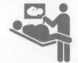

STRUCTURE OF ANTENATAL CARE

Whether your antenatal care is in the hospital or in the community, for an uncomplicated pregnancy the structure of your appointments will be approximately the same. Traditionally, you were seen every four weeks until you were 28 weeks pregnant (28 weeks' gestation), then every fortnight until 36 weeks' gestation, then weekly until the baby is born. The National Institute for Clinical Excellence has recently introduced new guidelines for the number and structure of appointments for antenatal care, where fewer appointments are generally needed.

If this is your first pregnancy you will have more appointments than if you have had a baby before. When a pregnancy is going well and there are no problems, a woman who is pregnant for the first time can expect to be seen on 10 occasions. If this is not your first pregnancy, you will have around seven appointments. Each appointment has specific purposes, which will be discussed in the relevant chapters. If you develop complications or problems, or even if you have concerns that you would like to discuss, you will be seen more often. Your doctor may decide that you require additional antenatal care, depending on your medical and obstetric history. This may be the case, for example, if you have had problems in a previous pregnancy, or if you have a chronic condition such as epilepsy or a cardiac condition. So, you may have a different number of appointments than other women you know, or even than during a previous pregnancy. (For more information about each antenatal appointment or scan, please refer to the relevant weeks.)

ANTENATAL APPOINTMENTS

10 weeks or earlier	The booking or first visit with various blood tests.
12 weeks	The first scan – a dating scan – and screening tests.
16 weeks	Antenatal appointment.
20 weeks	The second scan – an anomaly scan.
25 weeks (approx.)	Antenatal appointment if this is your first baby.
28 weeks	Antenatal appointment and blood tests.
31 weeks (approx.)	Antenatal appointment if this is your first baby.
34 weeks	Antenatal appointment.
36 weeks	Antenatal appointment.
38 weeks	Antenatal appointment.
40 weeks	Antenatal appointment if this is your first baby.
41 weeks	If you have not had your baby, a further antenatal appointment.
6 weeks after the baby is born	A postnatal check, generally carried out by your GP.

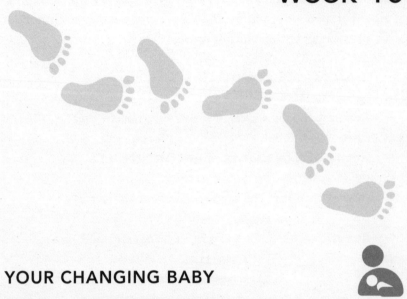

week 10

YOUR CHANGING BABY

Your baby's skeleton is continuing to develop, and although it is still made mainly from cartilage, bone will soon form. His muscles have now developed so he is able to move around, though as yet you still cannot feel these movements. His stomach continues to form and becomes connected to his mouth in which his taste buds are developing; the rest of the intestine is currently a long tube. His head is still big, about half the length of his body, and he has a large bulging forehead; the cells of his brain are still dividing rapidly.

His hands and feet become less like paddles as the fingers and toes begin to separate. Fingernail beds are developing; he even has finger pads on his fingers with his own fingerprints. As he now has a working mouth and jaw he starts to practise swallowing. The beginnings of a suckling reflex develop (he makes sucking movements if he touches his face) so he will be able to drink milk when he is born. Hair follicles are formed which will allow him to grow hair. He is approximately 3 centimetres long (just over an inch) and has doubled his weight again, to about 4 grams (0.14 ounces).

AMNIOTIC FLUID

Amniotic fluid is a clear, yellow-tinged liquid that surrounds the baby within the amniotic sac in your womb. It is produced from your placenta, your own circulation, the amniotic membranes and by the baby's urine. The amount of amniotic fluid produced gradually increases throughout the first two trimesters, reaching a peak at about Week 34.

It has various roles, including helping your baby's lungs and kidneys to develop. As your baby develops he will start to swallow the fluid. This will then be processed by his kidneys to produce urine, which he will urinate out into the fluid before starting the cycle again. He also breathes in some amniotic fluid and excretes it again via his lungs. It also has a role in helping your baby move – think about how easy it is to move in water as the water supports your weight.

The temperature of the amniotic fluid is 37.5°C, slightly higher than your body temperature. As your baby is not yet able to control his body temperature, the fluid helps keep him warm. It also acts as a cushion, protecting your baby from any bumps to your stomach, and may have a role in protecting him from infection.

Some of your baby's skin cells will be shed into the fluid, so a sample can be collected during amniocentesis to test your baby for various conditions (for more information see page 93).

Oligohydramnios is a condition where there is not enough amniotic fluid; polyhydramnios is where there is too much amniotic fluid. If your doctor or midwife is concerned that your bump is smaller or larger than expected you will be referred for an ultrasound scan where the amount of amniotic fluid can be measured. Causes of oligohydramnios include leaking membranes (your waters are leaking) and causes of polyhydramnios include diabetes.

YOUR CHANGING BODY

Your womb has now increased to approximately the size of an orange. You may have noticed changes in your skin, as high levels of progesterone may make it feel dry or spottier than normal. The veins under your skin may be more visible than usual because they have dilated to cope with the increased blood supply to the skin. Some women develop visible small blood vessels in the skin of their upper arms and chest; these spider naevi look like small spidery red lines, often in a star shape, and again are due to oestrogen making your blood vessels dilate. There is no point treating these visible vessels with creams as they tend not to work, and these lines generally fade after pregnancy.

'I keep getting pains. Is everything still okay?'

Many women have abdominal aches and pains throughout pregnancy. Women may describe these pains differently as pain is subjective, and different women will feel things differently. For some women these pains may feel like muscle aches; for others they may feel like sharp twinges. The majority of these pains are not a cause for concern, but if you have cramping pain associated with blood, severe pain or pain that doesn't go away, visit your doctor for investigation.

All the ligaments, muscles and connective tissues in your pelvis have to stretch to accommodate your growing uterus. Hormones such as relaxin help your connective tissues relax and stretch. As a result of all this stretching you may experience some abdominal aches or discomfort during your pregnancy, which can also be called round ligament pain.

'At first, every time I had a twinge in my tummy I thought it meant something was going wrong and I started panicking ... and I've been getting lots of aches and twinges so I spent a lot of time panicking! Since I was told that it is okay to get some aches, that it is just everything stretching, I've calmed down a lot. Now, when it happens I consider it a reminder of how wonderful my body is to be able to change and expand to make room for my baby.' Sonia, 36

YOGA AND RELAXATION TECHNIQUES

Pregnancy is a great time to start, or continue, yoga. Pick an antenatal or pregnancy yoga class or DVD; these are generally gentler and designed specifically for the needs and changing bodies of pregnant women. Yoga helps you to focus on and be aware of your body, and increases your strength and flexibility. It can also help to boost your energy levels and improve and maintain your posture. Relaxation is an important part of yoga, and these techniques will be helpful through pregnancy, labour and beyond. During pregnancy, avoid positions that put pressure on your bump, and don't overstretch yourself. Start by doing three repetitions of each pose; you can gradually increase the number of repetitions if you feel able.

When trying any relaxation technique make sure you find a quiet place and pick a time when you will not be disturbed and will be able to focus on yourself. Find a comfortable position, though keep your spine straight (for example sitting upright on a chair with your feet hip-width apart), and try to empty your mind and focus on your breathing. Counting to three or five as you inhale and exhale may help you slow and control your breathing. Let your thoughts drift in and out. You may choose to visualise that you are somewhere where you feel calm, relaxed and serene. Imagine using all your senses – for example, feel the heat of the sun while hearing the waves or breathing in crisp fresh air. Just five minutes spent focusing on yourself every day can help you feel relaxed and refreshed.

'WHERE SHOULD I HAVE MY BABY?'

You might now be considering your options about where to deliver your baby (for more information about labour itself, including pain relief, see 'Labour', pages 245–292). Options include having the baby in a hospital, in a midwifery-led unit or at home:

- **Hospitals** have doctors present and the facilities for emergency Caesareans and pain relief such as epidurals, but they can sometimes feel very medical and clinical.
- **Midwifery-led units** are suitable for low-risk births and may feel more informal and less clinical. Some forms of pain relief, such as

pethidine or gas and air, may be available, but not others, such as epidurals.

- **Home births** are advised only for low-risk pregnancies. You may be able to arrange a home birth with your community midwife or GP.

If you decide to deliver at home against your doctor's advice, a midwife from your local hospital still has a duty to attend your delivery. She cannot force you to go to hospital, though she may advise you to do so, as long as you fully understand the risks regarding staying at home.

At a home birth your midwife may be able to supply you with gas and air as pain relief, or she may be able to set up a birthing pool. In both midwifery-led units and home births, you can be transferred to your local hospital if problems do arise, or you decide that you want pain relief.

It is a good idea to visit the labour wards and maternity units at various hospitals and birthing centres in your area. Most maternity units offer tours of their labour wards, either in the evenings or at weekends. Taking a tour can help you get a feel for the atmosphere of the unit and attitudes of the staff. To arrange a tour, telephone the relevant labour ward or birthing centre.

Questions you might like to ask include:

- Will the same midwife be available throughout your labour or how long are the midwifery shifts?
- Will an anaesthetist always be available to administer epidurals?
- Are birthing pools or birthing balls available (for more information see page 252)?
- If you choose midwifery-led care, what are the emergency policies?
- What are their policies regarding induction of labour, instrumental deliveries and episiotomies (for more information see 'Labour', pages 245–292)?
- Are breastfeeding counsellors available?
- Are neonatal paediatricians available?
- Is there a neonatal intensive care facility?
- Is it possible to have a private room after the birth? How much would this cost?

There is no 'perfect' labour ward, just one that is best for you. For each woman this may be different, depending on your thoughts about pregnancy and labour. Ask around: your GP, family members or friends may have had experiences in certain places and may be able to advise you further. To pick a unit that fits your ideals, try to look beyond the wallpaper and carpet to the attitudes of the staff about pregnancy, labour and delivery.

'MY HUSBAND SAYS HE FEELS SICK IN THE MORNINGS. IS HE BEING SYMPATHETIC OR DOES HE JUST WANT ATTENTION?'

Some women report that their husband or partner also displays some of the symptoms of pregnancy. Very rarely they may develop a 'pregnancy bump' (called pseudocyesis) but more commonly symptoms include some weight gain, sickness or nausea or some emotional symptoms such as becoming more emotional or even developing a nesting instinct, rushing around doing home improvements before the baby comes. This is called Couvade syndrome and is thought to be becoming more prevalent as men get more involved in their partner's pregnancy. It is not known why this occurs; perhaps it is due to the psychological effect of preparing for a baby and watching the changes occurring in their partner, or it may be due to hormonal changes in men. The symptoms generally resolve after delivery.

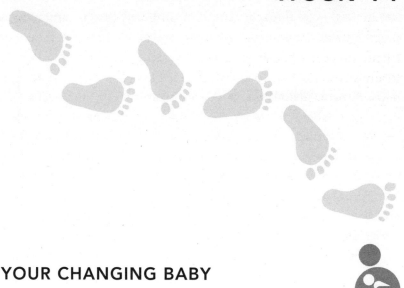

week 11

YOUR CHANGING BABY

Although you are only eleven weeks pregnant, approximately nine weeks from conception, by this stage all your baby's organs are fully formed. He now looks more like a human baby as opposed to a tadpole! He has fingers and toes, facial features and a tongue with taste buds. He will spend the next six months growing and maturing. His skeleton, previously made of cartilage, begins to harden into bone from this point, and he is moving in his pool of amniotic fluid, making both large and small movements such as flexing his fingers. His brain continues to develop, making thousands of connections and new cells.

Although the baby's sex is decided by its genes, this may not yet be visible on a scan. Boys are producing high levels of testosterone, which causes the development of male genitalia; without it, female genitalia form, the default state. The genital swelling will form into either a clitoris or a penis.

Your baby's skin is still very thin and transparent, and his blood vessels can be seen through it. His lungs are still very immature but his heart is beating away, up to approximately twice the speed of your own. He continues to swallow, and his intestine can now deal with the swallowed amniotic fluid. He is approximately 4 centimetres long (1½ inches) – less than the length of your little finger – and weighs about 7 grams (¼ ounce).

YOUR CHANGING BODY

Your breasts will have been changing rapidly and it can feel like they are growing exponentially! How much your breasts increase in the first trimester may depend on how large your breasts were before you became pregnant. If you had very small breasts the increase in size may be more obvious, and you may go up a few cup sizes. After the first trimester the breasts themselves tend to stop growing but you should still be measured regularly as you can get larger underneath the breasts and so need a bigger bra. Your breasts will then tend to increase in size during the last month or few weeks of pregnancy in preparation for breastfeeding. (For more information about bras in pregnancy see Week 6.)

'I feel so different and think about my baby and being pregnant all the time. To me it feels like there is a big sign over my head in huge red letters saying "I'm pregnant". It seems strange that other people don't know yet. Okay, I don't look any different yet but I'm pregnant and want to yell it from the rooftops. Next week I'm having my first scan. I can't wait to see my baby ... and tell everyone!' Marion, 26

'How much weight will I put on during my pregnancy?'

Appropriate weight gain in pregnancy is dependent on your starting weight – how much you weighed before you became pregnant. Body mass index (BMI) is a measure of your weight and is calculated by dividing your weight (in kilograms) by your height (in metres) squared, that is your height multiplied by your height again. A healthy BMI is between 20 and 25. If your BMI is below 20 you are considered underweight; if it is above 25 you are considered overweight.

Women who were underweight before they became pregnant will put on more weight than average during pregnancy, and women who were overweight previously will generally put on less weight during pregnancy. The average woman, of average height and weight, will gain approximately 10–15 kilograms (22–33 pounds or 1½–2½ stone) during pregnancy. If you are expecting twins or more you will put on more weight.

The weight gain is not steady throughout pregnancy. During the first trimester most women gain only a small amount of weight, perhaps a few pounds, or their weight may not change at all. In fact, many women find that they lose weight in the first few weeks of pregnancy due to vomiting or feeling nauseous and so not eating very much. From the second trimester onwards, until the last few weeks of pregnancy, you will gain weight weekly.

'I feel like I have a permanent runny nose!'

Many women notice that their nose feels stuffy or blocked during pregnancy, as if they permanently have a cold. Your ears can also feel blocked. You may find that you start to have a few streaks of blood when you blow your nose, or even a proper nosebleed. Your gums may also bleed, especially when you brush your teeth. This is a reflection of your increased blood volume – more blood is flowing to the mucus membranes in your nose, gums, ears and sinuses. Your pregnancy hormones can also make the inside of your nose swell slightly, which may mean that you start snoring!

LOOKING AFTER YOUR TEETH AND GUMS

Gums are more likely to bleed and/or become infected during pregnancy. This is due to a combination of the increased blood supply to the gums and the fact that your pregnancy hormones may soften them. It is important not to neglect your oral health as you may develop tooth decay or periodontal disease (gum infection/inflammation). This may even cause problems with your pregnancy, such as a low birth weight baby or premature labour.

Brush and floss your teeth regularly and make sure that you visit your dentist during pregnancy. You are entitled to free NHS dentistry while you are pregnant. Doctors and dentists try to avoid using X-rays while you are pregnant, but if your dentist recommends an X-ray they will protect your bump with a lead apron.

Most fillings, crowns and local anaesthetics are safe for use in pregnancy. If you require antibiotics your dentist will choose an appropriate option for pregnancy. It is currently advised that amalgam (silver) fillings are not inserted or replaced during pregnancy as they contain mercury. Other options, such as white fillings, may be used.

Mouthwashes are safe to use in pregnancy, though avoid mouthwashes that contain alcohol and try not to swallow them!

These symptoms generally last the whole of pregnancy and only resolve as your blood volume returns to normal in the six weeks after delivery. Avoid hot and dry atmospheres, or try putting a small bowl of water over a radiator to keep the atmosphere moist. If you get nosebleeds then apply pressure by pinching your nose (the soft part just above your nostrils) to help the blood clot; if this doesn't work you could try placing an ice pack or a packet of frozen peas over your nose. If the nosebleed doesn't stop within 30 minutes despite pressure and an ice pack, go to A&E. Regular and severe nosebleeds should be reported to your doctor.

THE BOOKING VISIT

You will be given an appointment for your booking visit around the end of the first trimester, either at the hospital or GP surgery with a doctor or midwife. Depending on your unit's policy, you will be sent an appointment by letter or given a telephone number to ring to arrange an appointment. This appointment may or may not be before your first scan, depending on your area.

The booking visit will probably be the longest antenatal appointment during your pregnancy and often takes approximately 30 minutes to an hour. Your doctor or midwife will ask you many detailed questions about your personal medical history, any previous pregnancies, your family history and your general health and wellbeing. You will also be asked about your social circumstances and any psychiatric history. It is important to answer as honestly and fully as you can, as from the answers you give your team will decide whether or not any extra investigations or special care will be needed during your pregnancy. Some of the questions may seem quite personal, though they are all relevant to your care and any information is confidential. The purpose of the booking visit is not just to gain information from you but to give you information about your pregnancy and the tests and care that you can expect.

Women are generally examined during their booking visit, though the extent of the examination may vary. Your blood pressure will be measured and you may be weighed. Your blood pressure will be taken at every antenatal appointment, so this first reading acts as a baseline and picks up if you already have high blood pressure. Depending on your doctor and medical history, a more thorough examination may be carried out to check out your general health.

You will be asked to give a urine sample at every antenatal appointment, which will be dipped and checked for protein. Normally there is no protein in the urine; if protein is found it could be a sign of an infection, so your sample will be sent off to the lab to be tested. Certain antibiotics are safe in pregnancy, and if a urine infection is found you will be treated with an appropriate antibiotic. Less commonly, protein in the urine signifies a condition of pregnancy called pre-eclampsia or a disease of the kidneys (if you are going to get pre-eclampsia it generally occurs in the third trimester; for more information see page 155). Therefore if protein is found in your urine it will always be investigated further, although in the majority of cases it is benign. At your booking appointment your urine sample will be sent to the lab irrespective of whether or not it contains protein. The urine is tested for infection as it is possible to have bacteria in your urine without experiencing any symptoms (asymptomatic bacteria). If this is the case you will be offered appropriate antibiotics to treat the infection.

Previously, women's urine was also checked to see if it contained glucose, which can be a sign of diabetes. During pregnancy your kidneys are working much harder than normal so some sugar may leak out into the urine. This occurs in up to about 50 per cent of pregnant women at some point in their pregnancy. However, this is not considered to be a reliable predictor of gestational diabetes (for more information see page 172) so most units no longer check the urine for glucose.

If you are under the age of 25 you will also be offered a test for chlamydia, a sexually transmitted disease common in young women, as part of the National Chlamydia Screening Programme.

This involves a urine test. If the test is positive, chlamydia can be treated with antibiotics.

You will also be offered blood tests at your booking appointment. These are routinely offered to all pregnant women. Further tests may be taken, depending on your medical history. Blood tests taken include:

- **Full blood count:** This looks at the numbers and types of cells in your blood. It also measures your haemoglobin level. If you are anaemic your haemoglobin level will be low and you may be advised to eat foods rich in iron, or take iron supplements.
- **Blood group and Rhesus status:** You will have one of four blood groups: A, B, AB or O. Within each group you will also be either Rhesus positive or negative. It is important that your antenatal team know your blood group in case you need a blood transfusion, so the correct blood can be given. If you are Rhesus negative you will be offered injections of a substance called anti-D at 28 weeks. Depending on the dose of the first injection, you may be given a second dose at 34 weeks and within 72 hours of delivery. This is because although you may be Rhesus negative your baby could still be Rhesus positive. If this is the case you may develop antibodies which can affect and damage your baby's blood, making it anaemic. Anti-D is a protein called an immunoglobulin which prevents this happening. You would also be given a further injection of anti-D if you have an amniocentesis or other procedure during pregnancy such as external cephalic version (ECV, see Week 35) or if you have any vaginal bleeding after 12 weeks. These injections prevent the formation of antibodies and prevent problems in this or subsequent pregnancies. If you are Rhesus positive you do not need anti-D injections.
- **Random blood glucose:** Some hospitals test a random blood glucose level; others test a level after a glucose load. For a random blood glucose test, no preparation or fasting is needed; for a glucose load test you will be given a certain amount of a sweet drink such as Lucozade to drink, and a blood test will be taken at

a set time after the drink. A glucose load shows how your body handles the sugar. Both of these tests aim to identify women who may have a problem with their blood sugar levels, and need a fasting blood glucose test or glucose tolerance test to check for diabetes in pregnancy. If you have a risk factor for developing gestational diabetes, such as being very overweight or a family history of diabetes, you may be offered a glucose tolerance test irrespective of this result (see Week 28).

- **Haemoglobinopathy screen (sickle cell disease and thalassaemia status):** All women are offered tests for the conditions sickle cell trait and thalassaemia. These blood tests look at the structure of the haemoglobin in your blood. If you have the condition, or if the tests show that you are a carrier for the condition, your partner will also be tested as there is a risk of passing these conditions on to your baby.

- **Immunity to rubella:** Infection with rubella (German measles) in pregnancy can cause problems in the baby such as brain damage and deafness. Most women are immune to rubella as they will have been vaccinated during childhood. Your blood is tested to check for your immunity to rubella. If you are non-immune you will be advised to avoid children or adults with unexplained fevers or rashes. The vaccine for rubella is not safe in pregnancy, but you will be offered the vaccine after delivery so that you will be immune in the future. Even if you have been vaccinated, immunity can disappear. Therefore, if you are found to be no longer immune, the vaccine can be offered in the postpartum period.

- **Hepatitis B and C:** Hepatitis B and C are viral infections affecting the liver. They can be spread by various methods including unprotected sex or sharing needles or other blood contact. If you have hepatitis B your baby is at risk of catching the infection during delivery. He will therefore be protected with an injection of antibody (IgG immunoglobulin) and/or then receive the hepatitis B vaccine, depending on the level of risk of infection. If you have risk factors for hepatitis C you will also be tested for this condition.

- **Syphilis:** Women are routinely screened for syphilis as this infection can cause severe damage to the developing foetus. If you are positive it is easily and quickly treated with penicillin.
- **Human immunodeficiency virus (HIV):** Women are offered a test for HIV as if they are an HIV carrier, taking medication during pregnancy can reduce the risk of transmitting the infection to the baby. Depending on the levels of the virus in your blood at the time of delivery your doctors may offer you a Caesarean, again to decrease the risk of transmission. The HIV virus is secreted in breast milk, so by not breastfeeding the risk of infecting the baby decreases. The baby may also be given medication to try to prevent it becoming infected. Many women are frightened about having an HIV test but if the result is positive there are many options to help both you and your baby.

The results of your blood tests will be sent to your antenatal team. In the hopefully unlikely event that there is a *serious* problem you may be contacted, though if all is well you will not be contacted but will receive these results during your next antenatal visit. Your antenatal team will produce a set of notes, which give details of your care and which are written in at every appointment. You will be given these notes at the next visit, at about 16 weeks. These are called 'hand-held' notes and you should bring them to every appointment or any extra visits.

YOGIC BREATHING

Learning how to control your breathing is fundamental to yoga. Yogic breathing will help you relax and may be useful during labour. Get comfortable and feel and observe your tummy as you breathe. Normally, as you inhale your abdomen expands, moving upwards and outwards, as you exhale your abdomen falls. Focus on this expansion, and notice that as you fill your abdomen you can then fill and expand your chest. As you exhale, feel your chest fall first and then your abdomen fall.

The movement of your abdomen correlates to your diaphragm moving downwards as you breathe. Your chest expanding correlates with the muscles in your ribs moving so you can hold more air. Breathing through your nose, while focusing on your breathing in this way, means that you will fill your lungs completely, oxygenate your blood, get rid of carbon dioxide and be able to use the full extent of your breath. As you focus on your breathing try to keep it slow and regular, like a wave: inhale, abdomen, chest, exhale, chest, abdomen – a continuous cycle. You can practise this breathing whenever you can, not just when doing yoga. You may find it relaxing and invigorating.

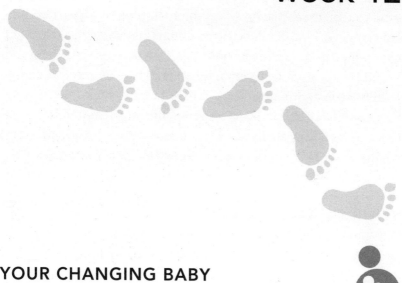

week 12

YOUR CHANGING BABY

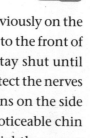

Your baby's face continues to change. His eyes were previously on the sides of his head; now they are moving closer together to the front of the face. Eyelids have formed, though his eyes will stay shut until approximately the seventh month of pregnancy to protect the nerves in the eyes. The ears also move to their correct positions on the side of his head, and your baby now has a profile with a noticeable chin and nose. His nose is button shaped and is turned up slightly so once he is born he can breathe when he is breastfeeding. He has vocal cords, and although he can't yet produce a sound, he may even be practising the movements of crying!

The intestine continues to develop, the pancreas matures and the liver produces bile, which will later help with digestion. Until now, the intestines were a tube wrapped around the umbilical cord, but by this stage the intestines have moved within his tummy. The kidneys are also working and a bladder has formed – the kidneys secrete urine into the bladder, which will eventually be urinated into the amniotic fluid. The baby then swallows this to start the whole process again.

As the brain continues to develop the baby becomes more responsive. He can feel touch on his body. He moves and squirms away from your finger when you prod your tummy. When you have your first scan, you might see that he moves when the probe is passed near him. Other reflexes have developed – for example, touching the palm of his hand would make his fingers close, just like a newborn clutching your finger! He is swimming in approximately 30ml of amniotic fluid. The fluid is a constant temperature, which helps to maintain his body temperature. It supports some of his weight and allows him to practise moving. He is now about 5 or 6 centimetres long (2–2½ inches) and weighs about 14 grams (½ ounce), about the size of a small plum.

YOUR CHANGING BODY

By the end of Week 12 your uterus will probably have grown from the size of an orange to the size of a grapefruit. At around this stage, between about 11 and 14 weeks of pregnancy, your womb will rise up out of your pelvis and into your abdomen, and your doctor will then be able to feel your womb by palpating your tummy.

In the majority of women the womb is flipped forwards (ante-verted) and simply grows upwards into the abdomen. In approximately 20 per cent of women the uterus is flipped backwards towards your back (retroverted). This generally does not cause any problems in pregnancy; in most cases, as the uterus grows it flips forwards so it can continue to increase in size into the abdomen. Occasionally, the womb does not flip forwards and can block the outflow from the bladder, causing pain and problems urinating. If you find that you are unable to pass urine, go to your doctor. In this rare circumstance a catheter is placed into your bladder to help you pass urine until your womb eventually flips forwards to continue growing.

12-WEEK DATING SCAN

You will be offered an ultrasound scan at approximately 12 weeks. This is often called the dating scan. You will be asked to lie down on a couch and a gel (often cold!) will be put on your stomach. The ultra-sonographer will use an ultrasound probe rubbed over your belly to get a picture of your baby. The scan itself should not be uncomfortable. The scanner will check the baby's heartbeat and then take a measurement from the top of the baby's head (crown) to its bottom (rump). This crown-rump length (CRL) is used as the foetus will probably have his legs curled up into his chest (the foetal position), so it would be difficult to get a length from his head to his feet. Your baby needs to be in profile (sideways on) to get the most accurate measurement, so if he is facing the wrong way you may be asked to wiggle your hips to try and get the baby to move.

Up until about the 12th week of pregnancy all babies grow at the same rate, irrespective of your and your partner's heights. The CRL measurement can therefore be used to calculate the age of the foetus and your expected delivery date. If this date differs from the expected delivery date calculated from your last period, the date from the scan will be used as it is considered to be more accurate as not all women have exactly a 28-day cycle and you may have ovulated earlier or later than is calculated from your dates. For example, you may have thought you were 12 weeks but be told you are 11 weeks pregnant. A further measurement may also be used in the calculation – the biparietal diameter (BPD), the distance between two bones on either side of the baby's head. After this point, the baby's length is no longer measured as a crown-rump length as this becomes less accurate as the baby can curl up or straighten out. Instead, alternative measures such as the BPD or length of the femur (thigh bone) can be used to calculate the age of the foetus and its growth. However, up until Week 20 an average crown-rump length, and after Week 20 an average crown-heel length, will be given in the book to give you an idea of how long your baby is. This scan also picks up whether or not you are carrying a single pregnancy, twins or even more! While for many women this is an exciting experience, it is also common to feel nervous or anxious – after all, you are meeting your baby for the first time.

You will be offered a picture of your baby during the scan. Some units charge for these photos, and the price can vary from approximately 25p to a few pounds for a printout. This dating scan is the first opportunity for you and your partner to actually see and meet your baby, a chance for bonding.

'Up until now I didn't really have an image in my mind. I don't think I truly understood that Suzy was actually growing a baby inside her. Of course I know she is pregnant and what that means but it is all happening to her, inside her ... But seeing it on the screen – the baby, my baby, our baby – looking like a real baby with legs and arms and everything brought it all home. We're having a baby. I'm going to be a dad!' Pete, 28

ANTENATAL SCREENING TESTS

Antenatal screening tests give a probability or likelihood of your baby being born with certain conditions. They are not diagnostic tests, which would give you a definitive answer as to whether or not your baby is affected. You will be offered various screening tests in your pregnancy, and as with any element of your antenatal care it is up to you whether or not you take the tests. Most babies are born healthy, but abnormalities may occur due to genetic factors, infections or other reasons.

Parents-to-be are understandably extremely concerned that their child is healthy and is developing normally, and even thinking about screening tests can cause some anxiety. The screening tests come quite rapidly, at the end of the first trimester, so you may like to think about or discuss them earlier. Before you take any screening or diagnostic test, think about what you would do if the test were positive; if a screening test gives you a high likelihood of your baby being born with a certain condition, would you have a more invasive diagnostic test such as amniocentesis, which has a small risk of miscarriage? If you did then have an amniocentesis and the baby was affected would you want to keep the baby? If you know that you would keep your baby no matter what, you may decide not to take the tests, or you may decide to take them so that you and your partner can be as emotionally prepared as possible. Screening tests commonly available are for Down's syndrome and neural tube defects such as spina bifida, a condition that can result in serious disability in the foetus.

All women are recommended to have the screening tests. You are at increased risk of having a pregnancy affected by a genetic condition if you have a previously affected child or pregnancy, are over 35 years old, or have a family history of a certain condition. You may also be at increased risk of having a baby with a certain condition if you know that you had an infection or took drugs that may harm the baby.

The National Institute for Clinical Excellence recommends that all women should be offered a 'combined test' to screen for Down's syndrome. The test is carried out between 11 and 14 weeks of pregnancy, generally at the time of your dating scan. At the scan the scanner will take a nuchal translucency measurement, which measures the fluid in the back of the baby's neck; the higher the measurement, the higher the risk of having a baby affected by Down's syndrome. Blood tests are then taken to measure the levels of various proteins in your blood (beta human chorionic gonadotrophin and pregnancy-associated plasma protein-A). The results of the blood tests, scan measurements and your age are calculated together to give a risk of Down's syndrome.

If you do not book for your antenatal care until after the point at which the combined test can be performed, you will be offered a triple or quadruple test, which can be performed between 15 and 20 weeks. Here it is not possible to measure the nuchal translucency, but the blood is tested for either three or four different substances and the results combined to give a risk of Down's syndrome. If you are carrying a multiple pregnancy the blood-screening tests also cannot be carried out as it is impossible to tell which baby the measured markers in your blood are coming from; the levels will be high as there is more than one baby, so in this case only the nuchal translucency measurement can be used.

Once the calculation has been made you will either be sent a letter or the results will be discussed with you at an antenatal appointment. The results are given as a risk: for a risk of 1 in 500, only 1 in 500 pregnancies will have a baby affected by the abnormality, or in more positive terms, 499 out of 500 pregnancies will be unaffected. Different units have different cut-off points as to what level is considered a positive test. This can be quite confusing. Say, for example, your unit has a cut-off point of 1 in 250. Whether your result is 1 in 260 or 1 in 2,500 you are considered screen negative, and therefore not necessarily advised to have further tests; and whether your risk is 1 in 240 or 1 in 30 the screen is positive and you may be offered further diagnostic tests.

You may disagree with what your doctors feel is a small risk and want to have further testing such as amniocentesis (for more information see Week 14). The tests are not perfect; in some cases a result is falsely high and in other cases falsely reassuring. Discuss your results with your partner and your antenatal team; screening tests can be confusing and it is important that you understand all your options.

If your screening tests are positive, after discussion with your antenatal team you may be offered further diagnostic tests, such as chorionic villus sampling (CVS) or amniocentesis. CVS can be performed after 10 weeks but is generally carried out between 11 and 14 weeks. Amniocentesis is performed after 15 weeks. These tests are diagnostic – they tell you whether or not your baby is affected by a condition (for more information see Week 14).

The vast majority of babies are born healthy. As with all parts of antenatal care, the aim of screening tests is to pick up those pregnancies which are at a higher risk of having a problem and then, after discussion with you, making choices about what further investigations and treatment, if any, are appropriate.

'I'M CRAVING PICKLES!'

During the first trimester you might notice that your sense of smell changes and becomes more sensitive. You may also suddenly develop strong aversions to certain foods, to the extent of being unable to tolerate even the smell. Food cravings, a well-talked-about topic, can also occur. Often, food aversions and cravings are associated with sickness and nausea, and doctors are not sure of the cause of these sudden changes in food preferences. It may be the body's way of obtaining certain substances it needs; a craving for salty foods may, for instance, be a way of replacing salts lost if you are being sick. Women often go off coffee, alcohol or cigarettes – perhaps this is to protect the baby from their harmful effects.

Even if you are eating only a limited diet, your baby will still be getting all its nutritional requirements from your body's reserves. However, if you are not able to drink fluids and are getting dehydrated, for example your urine is getting very concentrated, you should see your doctor. Hopefully you will feel better soon and will be able to return to a healthy diet; until then, keep your fluid intake up and just eat whatever you can manage.

YOGA

Keep practising your yogic breathing (see Week 11). You should use your yogic breathing whenever you do a yoga pose but also at other times when you want to relax. You and your partner can do a breathing technique together, sometimes called joined breathing. This helps you and your partner bond, both to each other and to your baby.

Your partner sits on the floor or bed with his legs open in front of him in a 'V' shape; he may want to lean against the headboard of the bed or something else to support his back. You then sit in between his legs with your back to him and lean back so he is supporting you. In this position he puts his hands on your lower abdomen, where your bump may be beginning to appear, and you either put your hands over his or on another part of your bump. He could put his head on your shoulder, or you could choose another position where you both can relax holding your bump. Once you are both comfortable in this position, focus on your breathing. You can use yogic breathing or just count your breaths. Inhale and exhale in unison; feel each other's breathing and your bump expanding beneath your hands as you inhale and enjoy the feeling of being close with each other and your baby.

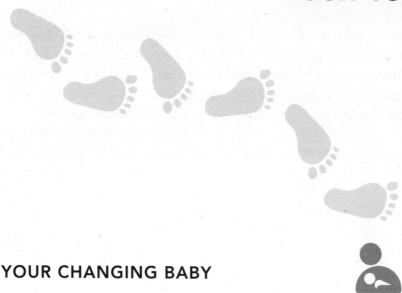

week 13

YOUR CHANGING BABY

By Week 13 your baby's neck has started to develop and lengthen. His head begins to straighten up instead of being curled into the chest and his chin has also formed; he looks more and more like a human baby. His intestines continue to develop to help him absorb nutrients from his food in the future. Arms and legs are getting longer and the bones are forming. He continues to move around, and although you can't feel it yet he may even respond by moving to or away from a prod in the stomach. He can open and close his mouth, stick out his tongue and has even become co-ordinated enough to suck his thumb. If the baby is a girl, her ovaries will already contain hundreds of thousands of eggs; this number will decrease by the time she is born, but these are the eggs from which she may have her own children. Boys' testicles contain the precursors to sperm but sperm is not yet produced.

On average your baby will be approximately 7.5 centimetres in length (3 inches) from crown to rump and weigh 25 grams (0.9 ounce). He will put on weight much faster from now on. In the first trimester the baby's organs develop; from the second trimester onwards your baby will grow and put on weight more rapidly.

THE PLACENTA

By Weeks 12–13 your placenta will be fully developed and functioning, though it will continue to grow in size throughout your pregnancy. Up until now your baby's needs were met by the yolk sac; now the placenta takes over and supplies your baby with oxygen and nutrients, and gets rid of its waste products. It also acts as a barrier for some infections and produces many hormones that adapt your body for pregnancy, labour and breastfeeding.

Before you were pregnant only 2 per cent of your blood volume went to your uterus; by the end of pregnancy, 25 per cent of your blood volume will supply your uterus and placenta. Your baby is connected to the placenta via the umbilical cord. This contains one vein, which carries blood containing oxygen and nutrients to the baby, and two arteries, which carry carbon dioxide and waste products back to the placenta.

The blood in your circulation does not mix with your baby's blood. The placenta can be thought of as a tree with lots of branches. These 'branches' bathe in the intervillous space which is filled with your blood. The membrane between your baby's blood and yours is extremely thin and allows oxygen, nutrients and waste products to pass between the two circulations. The cells of the placenta contain the same DNA as that in the cells of the baby, so a sample can be removed for genetic testing (for more information see Week 14).

YOUR CHANGING BODY

By the end of the first trimester your body will have undergone many physiological changes in order to accommodate your growing and developing baby. All your organs are working harder and therefore require more oxygen than before you were pregnant – about a fifth or 20 per cent more. Some of this increase goes to your breasts, heart, kidneys and skin, and about half goes to your womb, placenta and baby.

In order to achieve this you have produced more blood and your heart is pumping harder than normal. You also breathe in and out much more deeply than previously; with every inhalation you take in more oxygen, and with every exhalation you breathe out more carbon dioxide (a waste product). The hormone progesterone is involved with this adaptation. You may have noticed that you get out of breath more easily than normal or sometimes feel short of breath even if you have not exerted yourself. Throughout pregnancy you are effectively hyperventilating; although this sounds alarming it is a normal part of the changes your body is making to compensate for your pregnancy. When you exert yourself you have to breathe even more deeply to meet your further increased oxygen demands so you feel short of breath much more quickly than before your pregnancy.

'WHY DO I GET DIZZY?'

Feelings of dizziness are common in pregnancy. You may find that you feel dizzy or lightheaded when you change position or get up after sitting or lying down for a long period of time. This is because your blood has pooled in your legs as the weight of your womb presses on the blood vessels in your pelvis, making it harder for the blood to return to your heart. As you stand up quickly your body has to suddenly work against gravity to pump blood to your brain. The feelings of dizziness occur when, momentarily, not enough blood and therefore oxygen reaches your brain. Standing up slowly, or in stages from lying to sitting to standing, gives your body a chance to pump the blood up to your brain. This symptom can also occur if you are standing for too long – keeping moving ensures that your calf muscles help the blood return to your heart to be pumped out again around your body.

Low blood sugar

Dizziness can also be a symptom of low blood sugar levels. Other symptoms include feeling sweaty or clammy and, perhaps unsurprisingly, hungry. Dizziness due to low blood sugar levels can occur in any position, even when lying down. Women often have low blood sugar levels during the early stages of pregnancy, especially if they are finding it difficult to eat due to nausea. Even if you are feeling nauseous try to eat little snacks such as a piece of fruit, a cracker or a handful of nuts and seeds to prevent your blood sugar levels falling.

Although, in the majority of cases, these feelings of light-headedness or dizziness are nothing to worry about, if it is happening regularly and you are concerned, or if you have passed out or fainted, then visit your doctor to be checked over.

VEGETARIAN AND VEGAN DIETS IN PREGNANCY

During pregnancy it is important to ensure that your diet contains all the major food groups. Some diets are more likely to be deficient in certain vitamins and minerals. Vegetarians should ensure that they eat enough portions of dairy foods and eggs to meet all their nutritional needs. Vegans are more likely to have deficiencies in, for example, vitamin B12 because they do not eat any animal produce, and vitamin B12 deficiency can lead to anaemia. Vitamin B12 naturally occurs in animal products such as meat and dairy, and in yeast extracts such as Marmite. Breakfast cereals in the UK are often fortified with the vitamin. So, if you do not eat meat or dairy you may want to ensure that you eat fortified cereals. If you are concerned talk to your doctor who may advise B12 supplements during your pregnancy.

Protein is made up of substances called amino acids, just as carbohydrates are made up of a combination of sugars. Some of these amino acids have to be obtained from your diet (essential amino acids), while your body can make other amino acids from those which you eat. These amino acids are then used in many processes in the body, such as to repair organs or build muscle. Meat, fish, poultry, eggs and dairy products contain all the essential amino acids. Pulses, soya, nuts and tofu also contain amino acids but you need to eat a combination of these substances to obtain all the different types of amino acids that your body requires. If you are vegan, you will need to ensure that you eat different and varied protein sources, such as using different types of beans and tofu in a stew, so that your protein needs will be met.

EXERCISE IN THE SECOND TRIMESTER

Exercise is safe during pregnancy though you may have to begin to make compensations for your bump by this stage. You may have more energy than in the first trimester and feel better able to exercise. As your bump grows it affects your centre of gravity and therefore your balance. Sports requiring balance and which may lead to falls, such as horse riding or skiing, will become progressively more difficult and risky, and should be avoided as your pregnancy continues.

The hormones of pregnancy make your ligaments and tendons relax. This, combined with the weight of your bump, means that injuries are more likely in high-impact sports such as running or jogging. Many sports are suitable in pregnancy, such as swimming. Antenatal yoga or Pilates classes are more relaxing and gentle, as well as strengthening; aimed specifically at pregnant women, the exercises used will be possible with a bump. Finally, remember that exercise and being active can take many forms, such as walking up the stairs, carrying your shopping or walking instead of taking the car or bus. It all counts!

TELLING PEOPLE YOU ARE PREGNANT

You may have already told people that you are pregnant or you may have decided to wait until after your dating scan. By this point in your pregnancy the risk of miscarriage has fallen significantly, and many women now feel able and ready to tell their news. Of course, if you don't feel ready you do not have to tell, but in a few weeks' time you will start to show and you may not be able to hide it for much longer.

Many women and their partners are concerned about how others will react to the news that they are having a baby. You may have a friend or family member who is having difficulty getting or staying pregnant, and may be worried how they will take your news. Your pregnancy will bring changes, not just to your lives but to those of your family too. Your mother becomes a grandmother (or a grandmother again); your father a grandfather; your aunts and uncles become great aunts and uncles; and your siblings, aunts and uncles. Most people will be overjoyed and excited for you. People who are having difficulties may be sad about their own problems but can still be happy for you. It may be better to tell people face to face rather than let them guess or hear from someone else.

You may notice that some of your relationships and friendships change during your pregnancy and afterwards. Some of your friends may find it difficult to understand as you develop a new set of priorities, and you may find yourself closer to other women who are pregnant or who have young children. The majority of people will hopefully be delighted with the news of your pregnancy.

'She's pregnant, pregnant! It feels like I've been waiting so long but now I'm going to be a grandma. My little girl actually having a baby. Okay, while it makes me feel old – and the thought of being called "Nan" or "Gran" makes me want to throw some knitting needles at someone – I am so excited. I can't wait to be able to share this with her, and soon there'll be another little warm, sweet-smelling baby to coo over, and of course the advantage of being the grandma is if it cries I get to give it back!' Sandra, 56

'You're going to be a big brother!'

How and when you tell your children that you are expecting a new baby will probably depend on how old they are and how much they can understand. An eight year old may have lots of questions, while an 18 month old may notice that you have a bump but find it hard to understand what it means. You may wish to tell your child that you are having a baby before or around the time you tell other people, family and friends so that they understand what everyone else is talking about and don't feel there are secrets, or accidentally hear the news from someone else.

Children may be apprehensive about the unknown. They may say things like 'I don't want a new baby', or ask the same questions over and over again. Try and be patient and gently explain, using language they can understand, that there is a baby growing in your tummy. Try to make them feel special. You may be able to start giving them special big brother or sister jobs from an early stage, such as picking a new teddy for the baby or allowing them time to stroke your bump. Even if your child is too young to understand what your expanding bump means, they will pick up on your smiles and relaxed and happy body language as you talk about the baby.

Many parents buy a gift to give to the older child on the new baby's arrival, saying it is either from themselves or from the baby. The idea is that your other child associates the new baby with the excitement and pleasure of a gift. Be open and keep talking about the new baby and how happy you all are about the baby coming, so hopefully your child will become happy and excited too!

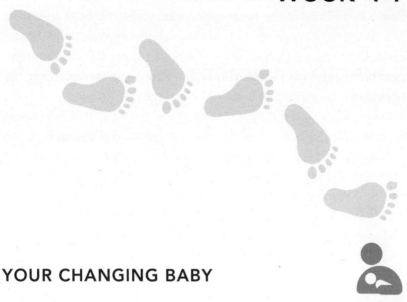

week 14

YOUR CHANGING BABY

Your baby can now practise breathing. He does not actually breathe as he gets his oxygen from your blood via the umbilical cord but he practises the movements that are involved, which become so important once he is born. He also practises moving in general – his movements will gradually become less jerky and more controlled as the connections between his brain and muscles and joints continue to develop. He can even make different facial expressions such as frowning or squinting.

Although his head is still large his body is beginning to catch up, making him slightly more in proportion, though he will have a proportionally large head even after he is born. The sex hormones continue to influence the development of male or female genitals. In girls, the ovaries move downwards from the abdomen into the pelvis; in boys the testes continue to develop, though they are still in the abdomen, and a prostate gland forms.

Hair grows on his head and eyebrows but also all over his body. The hair on his body is very fine, soft and downy, and is called lanugo hair. Lanugo hair protects your baby's skin from the effects of being constantly immersed in water; most or all of it is generally shed before birth. On average he measures 9 centimetres in length (3½ inches) from crown to rump and weighs approximately 43 grams (1½ ounces).

YOUR CHANGING BODY

By Week 14 of your pregnancy your uterus will have increased in size dramatically: it is now the size of a small melon and can be felt through your abdomen. Around this stage you may begin to 'show', that is you will develop a little bump and it will become more obvious that you are pregnant. Women who have been pregnant before tend to show earlier than those having their first baby. This is because their stomach muscles have already been stretched during a previous pregnancy and so stretch more easily.

'Finally, I'm hungry again!'

By the beginning of the second trimester the majority of women are beginning to feel better. As the nausea recedes you may find your appetite returning to normal and some of your food aversions may disappear. You may also find that the fatigue and exhaustion you might have felt in the first trimester subsides. All in all, many women feel back to their normal selves by this stage, or even better than before with lots of energy. If you are still feeling nauseous, don't worry, as it is still normal for some women to feel sick. This generally passes soon, often by Week 16, though there are a few women who feel nauseous throughout their pregnancy.

THE PELVIC FLOOR

The pelvic floor refers to the muscles that support your bladder, bowel and womb. It is like a sling or hammock running from your pubic bone at the front to your spine at the back. The muscles surround your vagina, urethra (tube where the urine comes out) and

PELVIC FLOOR EXERCISES

To find your pelvic floor muscles imagine going to the toilet and trying to stop urinating midway. The muscles you are tightening to stop the flow are your pelvic floor. You may want to try these exercises while you are urinating to be sure that you are identifying the correct muscle. However, don't stop urinating halfway through regularly as you want to be sure that you fully empty your bladder.

- Lift and tighten these muscles as much as you can and hold for 10 seconds. Repeat this exercise 10 times.
- Lift and tighten the muscles faster, 10 times again, but this time holding for only a second or a count of three.
- Imagine that your pelvic floor is like an elevator. Lift and tighten the muscles in three stages as if it were going up and stopping at three floors, then relax down in one smooth controlled action and repeat 10 times.
- Finally, do the last exercise in reverse: lift up and tighten in one smooth motion and then relax in three stages, like an elevator going down and stopping on three floors. Again, repeat 10 times.

Initially you may find it difficult to carry out these exercises for the 10 repetitions, or may even find it hard to locate your pelvic floor muscles. If you practise every day, they will get easier to perform, and hopefully should prevent you having any long-term problems.

anus. If these muscles become lax and have poor tone the hammock sags and can cause problems such as stress incontinence (leaking urine when you cough or sneeze).

Being pregnant puts pressure on your pelvic floor; this, combined with pushing during labour, can decrease the tone in your pelvic floor muscles. In order to prevent this loss of tone it is important to exercise your pelvic floor muscles daily, during pregnancy and afterwards. You should do them even if you have a Caesarean, as there has still been extra pressure on your pelvic floor during the pregnancy due to the weight of your bump.

Doing your pelvic floor exercises should be part of your daily routine throughout your pregnancy and beyond. You can start them at any stage and should do them daily, even when you are not pregnant! Think of something you do every day, such as watching the news or doing the washing up, and do your pelvic floor exercises while you carry out this activity. As it is not possible for anyone else to tell that you are doing these exercises you can do them anywhere, such as on your bus journey.

OTHER ANTENATAL TESTS

You will have been offered screening tests earlier in your pregnancy: blood tests and as part of your dating scan. Depending on the results of these and/or your past medical history, if there is a high risk of particular conditions you may be offered further tests such as chorionic villus sampling (CVS) or amniocentesis. These tests aim to be diagnostic, that is they don't give you a risk of a condition; rather they tell you whether or not your baby is affected by a certain condition. For example, if your screening tests showed a high chance that your baby had Down's syndrome, the cells obtained during one of the tests described below would be tested for Down's syndrome; if you know you are at risk of passing on a genetic condition, such as cystic fibrosis, the cells could be tested for that particular disease.

The test does not tell you about every possible disease, only the specific one of which your baby may be at a higher risk. You don't need to have both tests: one or other will give you a definitive answer. Which test is offered depends on how far along in your pregnancy you are. Each test carries a small risk of miscarriage; this is higher for CVS than amniocentesis, though CVS can be performed at an earlier stage of pregnancy. The length of time you have to wait for the results depends on the condition for which you are testing; the labs will get the results to you as quickly as possible.

It can be very difficult to decide whether or not to have a diagnostic test, or what to do if the result is positive. You will be offered counselling to discuss any questions you may have. There are no rights or wrongs, and there is no definite course of action; each woman or couple will make a decision that feels best for them, and shouldn't feel pressured by family, friends or professionals.

Chorionic villus sampling (CVS)

CVS can be performed after 10 weeks. Here a needle is inserted into the uterus under the guidance of ultrasound and a tiny amount of tissue is obtained from the placenta. Cells from the placenta contain the same DNA as your baby and can be tested for conditions such as Down's syndrome. The advantage of CVS is that it can be performed very early in pregnancy but it does have a risk of miscarriage of approximately 2 per cent. There is also a risk of introducing an infection into the womb, though precautions are taken to prevent this occurring. You do not need to have bed rest after the test, but for the first 24 hours it is advisable to avoid any heavy lifting, running or major exercise.

Amniocentesis

Amniocentesis is generally performed after 15 weeks. Again, using ultrasound as a guide, a needle is inserted into the uterus through your bump and a sample of amniotic fluid taken. The baby sheds skin cells into the amniotic fluid, which can then be examined to see if the baby is affected by a condition. The risk of miscarriage is lower than with CVS (approximately 1 per cent), but as it is performed later in pregnancy it may affect any decision you make if you're told your baby does have a condition. As with CVS, there is a risk of introducing an infection into the womb, but the procedure is performed in a sterile manner to try and prevent this from occurring. Again, you don't need bed rest but should take it easy, so no heavy lifting or exercise for the first 24 hours after the test.

Multiple pregnancies and diagnostic tests

As mentioned in Week 12, only the nuchal translucency test can be used as a screening test in multiple pregnancies. However, both CVS and amniocentesis can be carried out. If twins, triplets or more share one amniotic sac and placenta, they are identical and as such will have identical genes, so the procedure is carried out as described

'We were advised to have CVS as we had had a stillborn child affected by a genetic condition. We agreed that it was the right thing to do but it was still really scary. The actual procedure was fine; it was just the waiting afterwards. Will it be okay? Will I be the lucky one who miscarries a healthy baby? The waiting felt endless, though everyone was as nice and supportive as they could be. Getting the test results was like waiting for school exam results but worse! Thankfully, everything is fine with the baby. Now we are so glad we had it because we can relax. I can really start to enjoy my pregnancy and the thought of a healthy baby.' Roshni, 37

above. The answer from one sample will apply to each of the babies. If the twins, or more, don't share the same sac then it is extremely important that the cells are obtained from each sac or placenta and are not mixed up. This is not always easy and it may not be possible to obtain a sample from each foetus. The risks of miscarriage associated with these tests are higher with multiple pregnancies: approximately 4 per cent for CVS and 3 per cent for amniocentesis.

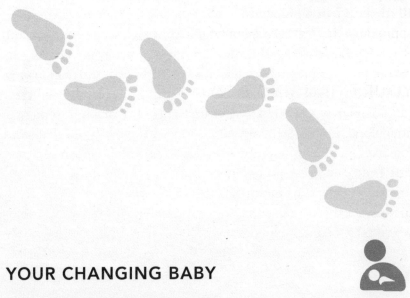

week 15

YOUR CHANGING BABY

Your baby's arms and legs have grown so much that his body is now longer than his head, so he looks more like a human baby. His bones continue to calcify and harden and his bone marrow develops – eventually it will make blood cells. His ears are now in their correct place on either side of his head. The bones of the inner ear also begin to harden so around this point in your pregnancy your baby will start to hear. Prior to hearing he may have been able to feel the vibrations of your heartbeat or your voice but now he can hear noises. It is noisy inside your womb; he will hear your heartbeat, the blood rushing through your veins, your food digesting. As his hearing improves he will be able to hear your voice and sounds from outside the womb. When he is born he will be able to recognise your voice, having spent so many weeks hearing it from inside the womb.

The bones of his face continue to develop, giving him cheekbones. He is shedding skin cells into the amniotic fluid, enough to be picked up on amniocentesis. He continues to practise moving, trying more intricate movements such as making a fist. As he practises breathing he may even get the hiccups; later in your pregnancy you may be able to feel when he has the hiccups. He is on average 10–11 centimetres (4 inches) long from crown to rump and weighs approximately 70 grams (2½ ounces).

YOUR CHANGING BODY

Your blood volume has increased to supply enough blood, and therefore oxygen, glucose and nutrients, to your baby and organs. In the first trimester, the liquid component of your blood, the plasma, increased. Now the amount of red blood cells in your blood also increases; otherwise your blood would become too dilute and you would get anaemic. About one quarter of your blood supply now goes to your womb and therefore your baby and placenta. Your heart continues to increase its output – the amount of blood it pumps out with each heartbeat – and the hormone progesterone relaxes your blood vessels so that they can cope with this increased blood volume without raising your blood pressure.

'My clothes don't fit!'

By around the 15th week of pregnancy most women have developed a little bump and are beginning to 'show', so it is no longer possible to hide the fact that you are pregnant. If your clothes no longer fit you properly, you may be able to wear them for a little longer with the help of elasticated waists and fabric or button expanders. Expanders are pieces of elastic or stretchy fabric that attach to your buttons and allow you to wear clothes that no longer do up. You may decide to put off buying maternity clothes until you are bigger. If you do decide to go shopping, look for clothes that will grow with you, such as elasticated waists or waists that fit under your bump and may have a support band on top.

TATTOOS AND PIERCINGS

If you have tattoos on your abdomen the designs will become stretched as your bump grows. Navel rings or bars should be removed as they may become uncomfortable and difficult to remove later as your bump expands and your belly button may protrude.

DIET IN THE SECOND TRIMESTER

As the nausea and fatigue of the first trimester subside you should find that your appetite returns. Try to remember to eat healthily and not to excess, though this is the trimester in which you will probably enjoy your food the most as you are not plagued by nausea or symptoms that become common in the third trimester, such as indigestion. Balance your meals and snacks to ensure that you are meeting all your nutritional requirements, and make sure that you are drinking enough fluids during the day. For healthy snacks try:

- hummus or guacamole with crudités
- nuts and seeds
- a juice smoothie packed with yoghurt, bananas and other fruit

If you fancy something a little bit more naughty try some granola (a combination of oats, nuts and fruit sweetened with honey) or popcorn, though it should be plain, not drenched in salt, butter, sugar or toffee!

'It is such a nice sensation to feel hungry again, and to enjoy eating without feeling sick all the time! My bump has appeared and my trousers are tight! I keep patting it, small though it is, and put my hands on my tummy like I've seen other pregnant women do. My bump may only be small at the moment but I'm still proud of it!'
Nisha, 23

ANTENATAL CLASSES

You may want to think about booking an antenatal class. Although you won't attend classes until the end of the second or beginning of the third trimester they do get booked up far in advance. Antenatal classes have many roles, including informing you about pregnancy, labour and life with a newborn, but are also important for enabling you to meet other people who are having babies. Classes may be arranged through your hospital, midwife or birthing unit. The National Childbirth Trust (NCT) also runs classes, and other privately run courses are available. Classes can range in price from nothing at all to several hundred pounds.

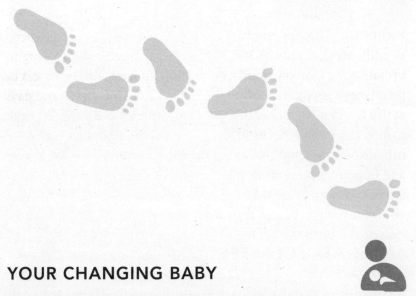

week 16

YOUR CHANGING BABY

Your baby continues to practise moving. By now he can control his limbs enough to kick or grasp his umbilical cord. He has lots of room to move around in, and the amniotic fluid dampens down your sensations of his movements. As he gets bigger he will kick harder, creating more movement in the fluid or even kicking the wall of your uterus, and you will be able to feel it.

He continues to practise breathing movements and now inhales and exhales amniotic fluid, which helps his lungs to mature. Although his voice box is fully formed he cannot make sounds as his windpipe is full of amniotic fluid; after birth the windpipe will contain air, so his vocal cords can vibrate to create noise. His brain and nervous system continue developing and maturing, allowing the formation of new reflexes such as the rooting reflex; this means that he will turn his head if you stroke his cheek to search for a nipple and therefore milk. The downy hair on his body protects him from the amniotic fluid and also helps regulate his body temperature. He measures approximately 11.5 centimetres (4½ inches) from crown to rump and weighs 100 grams (3½ ounces), about the size of a pear, and will approximately double his weight over the next few weeks.

YOUR CHANGING BODY

Up until now the amount of blood flowing to your kidneys has been steadily increasing, which is why you may have been needing to urinate more than previously. From approximately the 16th week of pregnancy the blood supply to the kidneys stops increasing and stays at this level, much higher than before pregnancy. Your kidneys work to filter and clean your blood and to control the amount of water you urinate out, thereby controlling the amount of water in your body and hopefully preventing you from becoming dehydrated. By this stage your kidneys are working up to 60 per cent harder than before you were pregnant, and they will continue having this increased capacity up until the last few weeks of pregnancy.

Although your kidneys are working so much harder than normal they cannot always meet the big demands on them and it is common for small amounts of sugar and protein to be leaked into your urine. At each antenatal appointment your urine will be checked for protein, and if it is present further tests will be carried out as it can signify other conditions such as a urine infection.

SKIN CHANGES AND STRETCH MARKS

You may have noticed that your skin has changed during pregnancy. The effects of pregnancy hormones generally improve your skin, although some women report that they have more spots than previously. Your nipples will have become darker, and the areola around the nipple will have become larger and darker in colour due to the effects of your hormones. Increased pigmentation in your skin means that any moles, freckles or even birthmarks can become darker.

A further effect of this pigmentation is that some women develop a 'mask of pregnancy', known as chloasma. On fair-skinned women this looks like tan-coloured dark patches over the cheeks and nose; on darker-skinned women these patches may look lighter than the normal skin tone.

Due to this increased pigmentation in your skin you may also notice that you tan more easily and quickly than normal during pregnancy. Of course, you should always wear high-factor sunscreen to protect your skin from the harmful and ageing long-term effects of sun exposure as well as burning. These changes are due to the hormones of pregnancy and tend to fade after delivery.

Stretch marks occur as your skin stretches to allow your bump to grow, and are due to tears in the collagen in your skin. They generally occur at times of rapid growth, such as during puberty or

ANTENATAL APPOINTMENT

At around this time in your pregnancy you will be offered an antenatal appointment. You will be sent an appointment or asked to phone to arrange one. The results of all the blood and screening tests taken earlier in your pregnancy will be discussed, and a plan set up for the rest of your antenatal care. You will be asked to give a urine test to check for protein; your blood pressure will be taken and you will be examined. Using a device called a Doppler, your midwife or doctor will check your baby's heartbeat, which you will be able to hear. This appointment is also an opportunity for you to ask questions or discuss any concerns you may have. At the 16-week check, or around this time, you should be given the details of where and when to attend for your next scan, the anomaly scan at approximately 20 weeks (for more information see Week 20).

pregnancy. The older you are during your pregnancy the more likely you are to get stretch marks as your skin becomes less elastic with age.

The majority of women will develop stretch marks during pregnancy. Initially these will look red or pink but with time will fade to a less obvious silvery colour, though they won't disappear entirely. Moisturising your skin may not prevent stretch marks appearing though it may help your skin stay soft and supple.

RELAXATION TECHNIQUES

Many women feel that they would like to spend some time looking after themselves during pregnancy, perhaps more than usual! Learning some relaxation techniques can help you relieve stress and focus on your body. These techniques, or some of the yoga poses described later (see page 123), may also help ease any aches or pains in pregnancy, or even help you relax during labour.

In a comfortable position, practise your breathing (see page 71). To help you relax further you could imagine a wave of heat passing through your body slowly, relaxing each muscle in turn. As the heat wave travels through you, imagine your limbs becoming heavy and relaxing into the floor or bed. Think about each part of your body in turn, every tiny muscle, each toe, each eyebrow ... Alternatively, you could tense and then relax each muscle group in turn – the action of tensing may make it easier to relax your muscles.

For some women it is easy to talk to, communicate with or bond with their bump and growing baby. Other women find it more difficult; they may feel uncomfortable or silly talking aloud or in their head to their baby, or may have had a previous experience that makes them uncomfortable doing so. Whether or not you are talking to your baby the bonding process will have already started; you are continually aware of the growing baby inside you and as such have already bonded. During a period of relaxation you might choose to focus on your growing baby, imagining what he looks like now or how he will look when he is born. Imagine your baby moving inside you, developing and growing.

'I like to lie quietly with my husband, with his head on my tummy, and gently talk about the baby, what it might be like to hold him, to know him. Or other times we just lie there, not talking at all, just breathing and being a family.' Cassie, 27

week 17

YOUR CHANGING BABY

As your baby's brain continues to develop he makes more and more connections, both between the cells in his brain and between his brain and body. For example, as he develops more connections to his muscles his movements become less jerky and more controlled.

His skeleton continues to harden, though there will still be more cartilage in it than in an adult as the bones need to stay more flexible. A sheath of a substance called myelin begins to develop around his spinal cord; this helps speed up the conduction of impulses along nerves. He also begins to create meconium, his first stool. This is a combination of bile salts and acid produced from the liver (which give it its greeny blackish colour), swallowed amniotic fluid and other cells from his intestine.

He still has a very fine layer of translucent skin and looks thin, but he is starting to lay down fat under his skin to keep him warm and for use as an energy supply after birth. His face continues to develop; his eyes now face forwards and are sensitive to light. He can detect light and dark through the translucent skin of his shut eyelids, which will remain closed until about 27 weeks.

Your placenta continues to grow and is now about 8 centimetres (3 inches) in length and 1 centimetre (½ inch) thick. There are approximately 200 millilitres (7 fluid ounces) of amniotic fluid, which helps your baby move and develop muscle tone as it supports his weight. He measures approximately 13 centimetres (5 inches) from crown to rump in length, and weighs about 140 grams (5 ounces), so he is about twice as big as he was two weeks ago.

YOUR CHANGING BODY

Your ovaries will be producing a hormone called relaxin. As the name suggests, this acts to relax and soften your ligaments, joints and other connective tissue to accommodate your growing womb, and to allow your baby to travel through your pelvis and birth canal during labour.

PALPITATIONS

Palpitations are the sensation of your heart beating, be it strongly, fast (racing), slowly or in an irregular rhythm such as missing a beat. They can occur whether or not you are pregnant, and can be due to various reasons, including anxiety. Palpitations are common in pregnancy, probably because your heart is working harder than previously due to the increased blood volume. However, they can be a sign of a cardiac condition so if you have very frequent or prolonged palpitations, or have shortness of breath, chest pain or dizziness with your palpitations or a history of a heart condition then do see your doctor.

This loosening of the joints means that you are more likely to develop backache (for more information see Weeks 24, 27 and 35). At the end of your pregnancy, relaxin is also involved in the process of cervical ripening, making your cervix soft and thin so that it can open and dilate in labour, ready for your baby to be born.

PLANNING A HOLIDAY? TRAVEL RULES

Now that you are hopefully feeling better and don't yet have a big bump, this is a great time to go on holiday. It is a good opportunity to spend quality time with your partner, and other children if you have them, without the stresses of everyday life.

Before you go

Make sure that you inform your travel insurance company that you are pregnant, and purchase a package that will cover you for any potential pregnancy-related problems. Some companies may not cover pregnancy after a certain stage so be sure to give them all the relevant information.

Take your hand-held notes with you so that if you do need to see a doctor they have all the relevant information they need. Check out the medical facilities near where you are staying, so that you know where they are if you need them.

Depending on where you are travelling to it may be recommended that you receive travel vaccines. Your local travel clinic will be able to inform you which vaccines are safe in pregnancy. It is advisable to avoid countries where malaria is prevalent. However, if you are travelling to a country where you will need to take medication to prevent you catching malaria, your travel clinic should be able to supply you with tablets that are safe in pregnancy. Even if you are taking malaria prophylaxis, take precautions such as wearing long trousers and sleeves in the evening so that less skin is exposed to get bitten.

Flying in pregnancy

Flying is safe in pregnancy. However, airlines generally do not let women fly after they are 34 weeks pregnant, though different airlines may have slightly different cut-off dates. This is because the airline does not want you to go into labour mid-flight! If you do have to travel after 34 weeks they may request a letter from your doctor.

Air travel has not been connected with miscarriage. If you have had miscarriages in the past, however, you may wish to avoid flying in the first trimester – not because it is risky but because you may not want to miscarry during a flight or in a different country.

Make sure that you walk around and move your leg muscles regularly, especially on long-haul flights. Pregnancy is a risk factor for developing blood clots – as is immobility, such as sitting down for long periods during flying – so moving around will decrease the risk. Flight stockings (up to the knee) put pressure on your lower legs, helping the blood flow back to your heart to prevent clots. It is also important to avoid dehydration so drink plenty of water (not caffeinated drinks). Even if you aren't flying but are sitting for a long period in a car or train there is a risk of developing blood clots so drink lots and try to keep moving.

Feeling the heat

If you are going somewhere hot and sunny remember that you may feel the heat more than usual when you are pregnant. Staying out of the sun, especially when it is at its hottest between midday and two in the afternoon, can help you keep cool. You will tan more easily than normal during your pregnancy due to the increased pigmentation in your skin. Wear sun cream and a hat and make sure that you drink plenty of bottled water to prevent dehydration.

Avoiding food poisoning

To avoid getting a holiday tummy or food poisoning, depending on where you are, drink only bottled water. Avoid ice in your drinks as ice is generally made with unbottled water, and peel all fruit and vegetables or wash them in bottled water. Most importantly, especially if you or someone in your party develops diarrhoea, make sure that you regularly wash your hands.

If you do get diarrhoea or vomiting, try and keep up your fluid intake to prevent dehydration. Drinking an oral rehydration solution such as Diarolyte, which has the correct balance of salts needed, can help. It can be bought over the counter and is safe in pregnancy, though be sure to add the correct amount of water when mixing it up. Anti-diarrhoeal medicines, such as Immodium, should be avoided during pregnancy. If you are unable to keep any fluids down and your urine is getting very concentrated, or you have not needed to pass urine for hours, then you should visit a doctor as you may be dehydrated and need fluids intravenously.

Holiday activities

For some people holidays are all about relaxing on a beach or by a pool; for others they are about sports, sightseeing or shopping. Whatever your plans you may notice that you need to have more toilet

'Okay, so I can't drink alcohol or go scuba diving, and my boobs don't fit into last year's bikini, but I feel fantastic, relaxed and content. I float in the pool wondering if it feels the same for my baby floating inside me and am constantly amazed – there are three of us on this holiday!' Sharon, 33

breaks than normal, and you may need to carry or buy a supply of little snacks.

Certain activities should be avoided while you are pregnant, including scuba diving, as the developing baby may not tolerate the changes in pressure and decompression needed. Snorkelling is not a problem as you are generally on the surface, breathing normal air, though whenever you are swimming in the sea be sure to stay in the areas which are monitored by a lifeguard, just in case you get into difficulties. Surfing, water-skiing and even water slides are best avoided, in case you fall straight on to your bump.

If you are proficient in a sport such as skiing, you may have been able to continue this in the first trimester. By now, though, your bump is getting larger and affecting your centre of gravity and balance, so sports such as this are best avoided.

Most importantly, relax and enjoy yourself!

week 18

YOUR CHANGING BABY

Your baby's lungs continue to develop and he practises opening his mouth as if to cry. He begins to produce vernix, a thick, white, sticky substance on his skin, which may still be present when he is born. Vernix protects his skin from the effects of being in the amniotic fluid for such a long period; without it he would be as wrinkly as if you had been sitting in a bath for too long. He continues to move around and can make more complex and intricate movements, from frowning to somersaults! He measures approximately 14–15 centimetres (5½–6 inches) from crown to rump and weighs about 200 grams (7 ounces).

YOUR CHANGING BODY

Your uterus continues to grow. By Week 18 of your pregnancy it has reached approximately the midpoint between your pubic bone and your navel (belly button). Your adrenal glands, found just above your kidneys, are involved in the production of a hormone called cortisol. From the end of the first trimester onwards the brain stimulates the adrenal glands, and also the placenta, to produce increased amounts of cortisol. This hormone affects most of your baby's organ systems and is very important in the development and maturation of his lungs. It may also be involved in producing stretch marks in your skin.

'It's getting hot in here!'

You may notice that you feel hotter than before you were pregnant, or that you are sweating more than usual. If it is the winter you may still be wearing thin summer clothes and not want the heating on, while if it is the summer, you may be feeling the effects of the heat as you get progressively heavier. This is a reflection of the increased blood volume in your body – as more blood is pumped to your skin, hot from the core of your body, you feel hotter. Sweating is one of the body's mechanisms of cooling down, so the hotter you feel, the more you will sweat. You may develop heat rash or sore spots from sweaty skin rubbing together, such as between your legs or under your breasts. Try to keep cool, avoid the midday sun and drink lots of water. Wearing layers of thin clothes means that you can peel off the layers as you feel hot.

'I am hot, hot, hot. I commend women who get pregnant and live in deserts and hot places. I think I would just have to lie down in a quiet room! It is winter and everyone is wrapped up in coats and hats, with woolly gloves and scarves wrapped around their necks, and then there is me, in a vest top, sweating and red in the face as I walk up the hill to work!' Belle, 31

BUYING NEW CLOTHES

As your bump continues to grow you will need to buy or borrow some clothes to wear at home and at work. You do not need to buy an entirely new wardrobe; remember you will only be wearing these

SEX IN THE SECOND TRIMESTER

Many women find that their libido returns or increases during the second trimester, probably because they are feeling better physically, and are less tired and nauseous. Remember, unless your doctor specifically tells you otherwise, sex is safe during pregnancy (see also 'Sex in the First Trimester', page 53).

As yet, your bump is probably not so large as to be getting in the way during intercourse, though as your pregnancy continues you may need to change or find new positions that do not put pressure on your abdomen, such as 'woman on top'. Often women report that they find sex more enjoyable and that it is easier to reach orgasm during pregnancy; this is probably due to the increased blood flow to your genitals. Many men will find your changing shape sexy and attractive, but if you don't feel up to sex there are many ways to stay connected and close, physically and emotionally, to your partner, that may not involve full sexual intercourse.

clothes for a few months. You may be able to borrow T-shirts or other items from your partner, but although they may be bigger than your own clothes they won't necessarily be cut to accommodate a bump!

Depending on the season in which you are pregnant you may be able to wear your own clothes for longer. For example, you may be comfortable in floaty tunic-style tops and skirts in the summer. Buying tops a few sizes bigger than normal is an option but there is a good choice of maternity wear available. You can buy clothes from maternity shops or concessions in high street shops, online or via catalogues. Browse charity shops for second-hand maternity clothes, or look out for sales of pre-owned maternity clothes organised by your local National Childbirth Trust.

The most important thing is that you are comfortable, so maternity clothes are often loose fitting, or made from soft stretchy fabrics which will show off your new shape. Maternity clothes are designed to expand with you. For example, tops are longer in the front than the back so when your bump takes up more room in the front, the front and back are the same length. Trousers and skirts can be bought with various waists. They can sit underneath your bump, on your bump (with an elastic waist, elastic inserts or expanding waist with buttons) or have an elastic or jersey panel that goes over your bump and expands with you.

Maternity tights can provide support for your bump and legs, and maternity knickers are available that go over or under your bump, though you may prefer to continue to wear your normal knickers that sit under your bump. You probably have already had to buy new bras (for more information see Week 6).

Remember all the times you bought clothes in the sales that you never wore, just because they were cheap? To prevent buying things that you won't wear, have a think about your daily life and the clothes you will need. For example, you may need a smart work wardrobe, lots of casuals or, if you are a regular swimmer, a maternity swimming costume. It may be easier to buy a couple of pairs of trousers or skirts and a few different tops that will go with both so that you can mix and match.

Once you have some outfits, think about accessories. Great jewellery or shoes can keep your often relatively small maternity wardrobe looking fresh. However, you may find that your feet swell as your pregnancy continues and you may not be able to squeeze into certain shoes. You may also find that you cannot wear high heels without being uncomfortable.

week 19

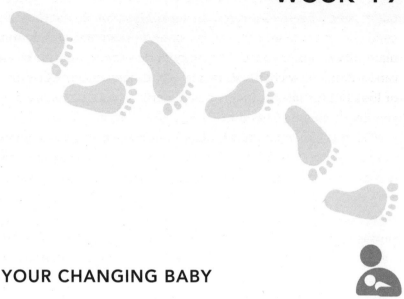

YOUR CHANGING BABY

Your baby's brain and nervous system have been developing extremely rapidly. Cells in the nervous system are becoming more specialised. His senses are developing: he can feel touch, for example, if you massage your tummy; he can hear; can respond to light and dark; has taste buds and the capacity for smell. Soon he will show you that he can hear by moving around to music or by jumping at loud noises, though you can't tell if he is moving to music because he likes it or because he wants you to turn it off! He may begin to grow hair on his head. His movements continue to become stronger and more co-ordinated, and soon you may be able to feel them. He measures approximately 15–16 centimetres (6 inches) from crown to rump and weighs about 240 grams (8½ ounces).

YOUR CHANGING BODY

As your baby, placenta, uterus and other organs continue to grow, they need even more blood so that they receive the oxygen and glucose they require. Your heart continues to increase the amount of blood it pumps out per beat, though your heart rate does not get much faster. Progesterone carries on making your blood vessels relax and dilate, decreasing their resistance and preventing your blood pressure from rising. In the later stages of pregnancy, from approximately Week 30, your blood vessels will not be able to dilate any further. The continuing increase in your blood volume means that your blood pressure will slowly begin to rise to your normal pre-pregnancy levels, but it should still not be high or increase suddenly.

Your metabolic rate is how efficient your body is at converting food into energy or stores of fat. During pregnancy, your metabolic rate increases. Your baby also has a metabolism. Both metabolisms create heat as they produce energy. Some of your increased blood volume goes to your skin; this helps your body get rid of some of this heat so it can maintain a constant temperature and prevent overheating.

'I THINK I FELT IT MOVE!'

Your baby has been moving around inside you for weeks but you won't have been able to feel the movements. At around 18–20 weeks of pregnancy you may begin to recognise these movements; the first time you do so is called 'quickening'. If you have been pregnant before you may notice these movements earlier as you know what you are expecting to feel.

You cannot feel movements earlier as in the early stages of pregnancy there is proportionally more room for the baby to move around. Kicks and stretching movements do not yet touch the sides of your womb, and any movements are cushioned by the amniotic fluid. As your baby gets bigger, his movements become stronger, creating larger ripples in the amniotic fluid. This then stimulates the nerves of your uterine walls and can be felt. As your pregnancy progresses there is less room for the baby to move around. You will feel movements more strongly or even see your bump move as he kicks the side of your womb.

Quickening can be difficult to recognise. These movements are often described as a fluttering sensation, or as if something were blowing bubbles inside you, or sometimes as if you had gas in your tummy. Initially you may not know these for what they are but as they persist and become more regular you may begin to recognise them. Don't worry if you haven't felt the baby move yet; some women feel the movements earlier than others. With time these movements become stronger and more definite, though it will still be a few weeks until your partner can feel them through your abdomen. The first time you feel the baby move can be special – you have been aware of your pregnancy for months but now you can actually feel the baby!

> 'I thought I felt something but that was three days ago and I haven't felt anything since. I can't wait to feel it, but almost as much I can't wait for Adam to be able to put his hand on my belly and feel a kick to remind us that baby's in there!' Sophie, 36

INCREASING YOUR FRUIT AND VEG INTAKE

We should all eat at least five portions of fruit and vegetables a day, though according to the Department of Health, the average person in the UK eats fewer than three portions daily. Aim for five portions as a minimum – you can have more! Eating fruit and vegetables may decrease your risk of developing cancer or having a stroke. They also provide fibre in your diet, which helps keep your bowels regular. This is even more relevant during pregnancy when constipation is common.

Any kind of fruit or vegetable counts – fresh, frozen, tinned, dried or juiced. Juice should be 100 per cent pure juice (not squash). No matter how much juice you drink per day it only counts as one portion as it does not contain much fibre and can be very sugary (so bad for your teeth). The sugars in fruit juice are fruit sugars, from the fruit itself, so even if the juice carton says 'no added sugar', the juice will still be sugary.

Some vegetables, such as peas, actually have more nutrients if they are frozen, as these vegetables leak their vitamins and minerals the longer they are sitting on the shelf; flash-freezing them soon after they have been picked means that they retain their nutrients. Try to avoid over-boiling your vegetables as the nutrients will leak out into the cooking water. Steaming is a healthy and tasty way of cooking vegetables, which helps retain their nutrients.

A portion of fruit is, for example:

- one apple or pear
- two satsumas
- half a grapefruit
- a good handful of grapes
- three dried apricots

For vegetables a portion is:

- 3 tablespoons of peas or cooked carrots
- one medium tomato (or seven cherry tomatoes)
- a small bowl of salad
- a medium-sized onion used as part of cooking, such as in a stir-fry or pasta sauce

Pulses such as haricot beans or lentils also count towards your five a day, though, like juice, no matter how much you eat they are only considered one portion as they don't contain the same range of nutrients as other vegetables. Unfortunately, potatoes do not count as they are classed as carbohydrates alongside other starchy foods such as rice or pasta.

Fruit and vegetables can be incorporated into every meal. This doesn't mean eating limp boiled vegetables! Try putting some fruit on your cereal, have a fruit juice or smoothie at breakfast or carry some dried fruit with you as a snack. Vegetables can be eaten cooked or raw: try having a salad with your lunch or crunchy crudités at snack time. Vegetables can be included in stews and casseroles or blended in sauces and soups. Desserts can be fruity, such as fresh or puréed cooked fruit in a yoghurt.

In total the amount of fruit and vegetables you eat should make up about one third of your diet. Try eating a range of different and brightly coloured fruit and vegetables daily. It's a good opportunity to experiment, and you might find something you didn't know you liked.

Taking vitamin and mineral supplements will not give the same effects as eating these foods. As long as you are eating a varied and healthy diet, the only vitamin supplements needed in pregnancy are folic acid (for the first trimester) and, for some groups of women, vitamin D (for more information see Weeks 1–4).

'I didn't realise how little fruit and veg I used to eat. I thought I ate plenty but when I actually worked it out I was lucky if I managed two or three portions. It was only during my pregnancy that I actually looked at what I ate. Now my family eats really healthily and, just as importantly, it actually tastes good!' Cathy, 31

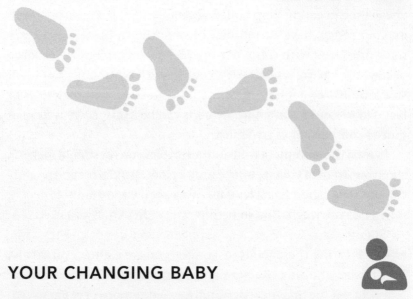

week 20

YOUR CHANGING BABY

Up until now your baby has been growing rapidly, both in length and weight. His growth begins to slow down from this point. His organs, such as his lungs, continue to mature.

At 20 weeks your placenta may lie low in your uterus; as your pregnancy continues and your uterus grows the site of the placenta often moves up and away from the cervix. The placenta is still growing and now weighs about 200 grams (7 ounces). You now have approximately 300 millilitres (10½ fluid ounces) of amniotic fluid.

At this point your baby measures around 16.5 centimetres (6½ inches) from crown to rump and 25.5 centimetres (10 inches) from crown to heel. The crown-heel measurement is not generally used during ultrasound scanning; instead other measurements such as femur (thigh bone) length and head measurements are taken to calculate age and growth if required. From this stage in the book the measurements are crown-heel lengths, simply to give you an idea of how long your baby is. He now weighs about 300 grams (10½ ounces).

WEIGHT GAIN IN PREGNANCY

On average, women gain approximately 0.5–1 kilogram
(1–2 pounds) per week during the second trimester. The
exact amount gained each week may vary – some
women gain weight steadily while others gain nothing
one week and then double the next. At the end of your
pregnancy weight gain slows down again.

The majority of this weight gain is not from fat.
Some is from the baby (the average baby weighs
approximately 3–4 kilograms or 6½–9 pounds),
placenta and amniotic fluid. Some is from the
increased size of your womb and breasts and extra
blood volume. On average, only 2.5 kilograms
(5½ pounds) is from fat. This is laid down so that you
have extra energy stores to meet the demands of
breastfeeding.

It is important to continue to eat healthily and not to
excess as if you lay down more fat than required it can
be difficult to lose it after giving birth. If you are
putting on excessive amounts of weight you will also
have an increased risk of developing gestational
diabetes (see page 172). Remember, your calorie
requirements increase only in the last trimester of
pregnancy, and then by only 200–300 kilocalories
(kcal) per day. The odd treat can be extremely
enjoyable, as long as it is in moderation.

YOUR CHANGING BODY

Halfway through your pregnancy, at Week 20, the top of your womb can be felt at your belly button. At each antenatal appointment from now on, your midwife or doctor will measure the distance between the top of your womb and your pubic bone – the symphyseal fundal height (SFH) – simply by feeling your tummy and using a measuring tape. This measurement approximately correlates with how far along in your pregnancy you are, with an accuracy of about 2 centimetres, as long as you are not pregnant with twins. So, at 30 weeks your SFH should measure between 28 and 32 centimetres. If you measure much bigger or smaller than expected you will probably be referred for an ultrasound scan. The scan will, among other things, measure the amount of amniotic fluid, as various conditions in both you and your baby can affect how much fluid you develop. If you are carrying twins or more you will be much bigger than if you were carrying one baby.

ANOMALY ULTRASOUND SCAN

By this stage in your pregnancy all your baby's organ systems are developed enough to be seen on ultrasound scan. During this scan, performed between 18 and 22 weeks, at approximately week 20, various measurements will be taken and your baby and womb examined to check that they are developing normally. In most cases the scan is normal; if there is a problem your team will discuss it with you and decide if any further investigations or treatments are needed.

Measurements taken include your baby's head, abdomen and thigh bone, and all the organs will be examined. Your placenta and level of amniotic fluid will also be checked. At this scan about one in five women will have a low-lying placenta; this will generally rise up as the pregnancy continues. If this is the case you will be offered a later scan at around 32–36 weeks of pregnancy (for more information see page 205). The scan is also an opportunity to see and bond with your baby and have another picture to take home.

BOY OR GIRL?

If the baby is lying in a position where its genitals can be seen, you may be able to find out the sex of your baby. Some hospitals do not disclose the sex as it can be difficult to see whether there is a penis or if the baby has just moved into a position where it cannot be seen.

'The difference from seeing my baby on the scan last time is huge. Now we could actually see its face with a little nose and mouth and ears! It has everything now and you can see it all working. They showed us the heart pumping away really quickly and it kicking its legs – it even brought up its hand like it was waving hello! It was so exciting but also really moving.' Shona, 28

YOGA

Many women find yoga helpful during pregnancy, not only for relaxation but also to keep them flexible and strong. As mentioned previously, you may wish to join a local class or follow a DVD at home (see Weeks 10, 11 and 12).

One of the most common yoga poses is 'tadasana' or 'mountain' pose. This is regularly used both before and after other poses, or on its own. The pose is supposed to help you become still and strong, yet powerful, like a mountain.

- Look straight ahead and stand with your feet hip-width apart.
- Feel your weight through your feet into the floor, using all of your feet from the heels to the toes.
- Your arms should hang straight down from your relaxed shoulders with your palms facing into your body.
- Try to use your yogic breathing while in this, or any, yoga pose (see Week 11).
- Imagine your spine lengthening as you breathe in. As you breathe out, feel the weight of your body being grounded into the floor. Feel the energy in your body, from your feet anchoring you to your fingers stretching to the floor.
- Focus on your breathing and body, being still but strong and relaxed.

A variation on this pose involves bringing your arms up and placing your palms together (as if in prayer) at chest level. As you inhale, using your abdomen and chest, open your arms. Sweep them down then up and outwards to a position where both arms are over your head, palms facing but not touching with fingers stretching to the sky. Feel your spine lengthening and the energy in your fingers as you stretch. Exhale and bring your arms back down to mountain pose. This pose helps the rib cage to lift and expand fully and so encourages you to use your breathing fully and warms up the body.

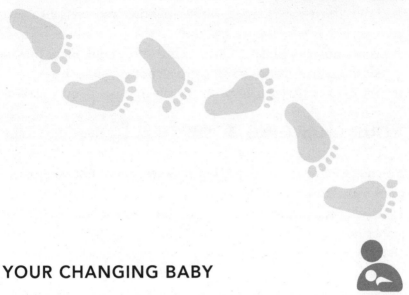

week 21

YOUR CHANGING BABY

By this week you may have felt the first flutterings of your baby moving, though they won't be strong enough to be felt by your partner for a few weeks. Don't worry if you can't feel anything yet; women describe feeling the first movements any time between about 16 and 24 weeks.

Your baby can now hear sounds both from inside your body and from the outside world. The sounds he hears are muffled by the amniotic fluid; imagine being submerged in water in a swimming pool with music playing or someone talking. He will recognise your voice and even types of music when he is born. If you have a particular piece of music that you enjoy, try lying down and relaxing when you listen to it; slow your breathing down and focus on you and your baby, or sway gently in time with the music. If you do this regularly you may find that your baby also begins to find that piece of music calming. This can continue after birth with your baby relaxing, or hopefully stopping crying, when the piece of music he recognises is played. Music can be relaxing to both you and your baby so tune in!

Although he gets his nutrition from the placenta, your baby continues to swallow amniotic fluid. He may get some sugars from the amniotic fluid, and his intestine is developed enough to process any swallowed sugars. Your baby's eyebrows and eyelashes have formed, as have the fingernails, though these will still be soft. He measures approximately 26.5–27 centimetres (10½ inches) from crown to heel and weighs about 360 grams (12¾ ounces).

YOUR CHANGING BODY

You might have noticed a dark line appearing on your tummy, from your belly button down to your pubic hair. This is called the linea nigra, and is another sign of the increased pigmentation in pregnancy (for more information see Week 16), though it does not appear in all women. The line marks the point at which your left and right stomach muscles used to meet; now they have to separate so that there is enough room for your bump to grow. This line can be very dark, hence its name, which literally means 'the black line'.

Rashes and itchy skin

Many women notice that their skin is getting dry, especially over their bump. As the skin on your abdomen stretches it gets thinner and may become dry and itchy. You may also notice dry patches on your arms and legs. Using a moisturiser should help soothe the itch and keep skin soft and supple.

The increased blood supply to your skin makes you feel hotter than normal so you may notice you are sweating more. Rashes can appear in creases such as under your breasts or in your groin where the skin is damp from sweat and rubs together. Heat rash can also appear due to blocked sweat glands. This looks like little red bumps in the skin and can be very itchy. Wear loose cotton clothing, try to stay out of the heat, and maintain good hygiene. A cool bath or shower may help with heat rash.

SEVERE GENERALISED ITCHING

If you notice that you have severe itching all over your body, which may include the palms of your hands and soles of your feet, inform your antenatal team. This is a symptom of an uncommon condition of pregnancy called obstetric cholestasis. This affects your liver, resulting in high levels of bile salts being deposited in the skin, causing the itching. The main risk of this condition is stillbirth. It is treated with medication. In later pregnancy, the baby may be induced early to prevent problems as the condition generally resolves itself after delivery.

MATERNITY RIGHTS AND BENEFITS

Every woman is entitled to maternity leave of up to a year, though not all of this will be paid leave. By law, your job must be kept open for you to return to, or your employer must offer you a job at a similar level. You cannot be sacked or made redundant simply for becoming pregnant. If you feel this has happened you can sue your employer for unfair dismissal.

You can find up-to-date information on maternity rights and benefits from:

- the Department for Work and Pensions (www.dwp.gov.uk)
- HM Revenue & Customs (www.hmrc.gov.uk)
- www.direct.gov.uk
- your local Jobcentre Plus

You will be able to find out about earning thresholds, eligibility for particular types of maternity pay and allowances, and values of and more details about each benefit including paternity pay, child benefit and tax credits.

Maternity leave

Statutory maternity leave is for 52 weeks (though you can return earlier) and you may be eligible for statutory maternity pay for 39 weeks of your leave. Maternity leave must be taken all in one block and can be started from 11 weeks before your expected due date. Your employer must also give you reasonable time off for any antenatal appointments or scans during your pregnancy.

If you fall ill during your pregnancy, even with a pregnancy-related condition, any leave required before 11 weeks prior to your due date will be considered sick leave. You can work right up to your due date, but if you have a pregnancy-related illness in the last four weeks of pregnancy that requires time off, your employer can insist you start your maternity leave from that date.

In order to take your maternity leave and claim maternity pay you must obtain a MAT B1 form from your midwife or GP and give this to your employer when or before you are 26 weeks pregnant. You must also give written notice at least 15 weeks before your expected delivery date of the date when you would like to start your maternity leave. If you change your mind about the date on which you would like to start your leave you must inform your employer in writing at least 28 days before you wish to start your leave in order to claim your statutory maternity pay. If you have your baby before you had aimed to start your maternity leave, your leave and benefits will commence on the day you give birth.

Statutory maternity pay

You will be entitled to statutory maternity pay (SMP) if you have been working for the same company for six months (26 weeks) by the date which is the 15th week before your expected due date and have been earning over a certain threshold (for more information, ask your employer if you are eligible). You can have been employed full- or part-time.

If these conditions apply you will be entitled to receive SMP for 39 weeks (nine months). For the first six weeks you will be paid 90 per cent of your average weekly salary and then basic SMP for the remaining 33 weeks of your maternity leave. You can then take an additional 13 weeks of unpaid leave, resulting in a total of one year's maternity leave. SMP is paid even if you do not plan to go back to work, or if you decide to go back to work and then change your mind.

Depending on your particular contract, you may have a more generous maternity payment package but SMP is a legal requirement and so is the least you can expect to be paid. If your contract does entitle you to more generous maternity payments then you may have to pay the extra money back if you decide not to return to work.

Maternity allowance

If you are not entitled to statutory maternity pay you may be able to receive maternity allowance. This may apply, for example, if you are

OTHER BENEFITS AND GRANTS

If you are not entitled to either statutory maternity pay or maternity allowance you may still be eligible for maternity incapacity benefit (payable for eight weeks in total) and/or a Sure Start maternity grant. For further information contact your Jobcentre Plus.

self-employed or have recently changed jobs (so have not been working for the same company for six months). To qualify you will need to have been in work (self-employed or employed) for at least 26 weeks in the 66 weeks before your expected delivery date, and to have earned over a certain threshold. If these conditions are met the Inland Revenue will then pay you 39 weeks (nine months) of maternity allowance. This allowance can be claimed from 11 weeks before the baby is due, though the latest date that you can start to claim is the day after your baby is born.

To claim, your employer should give you an SMP1 form if you are not entitled to statutory maternity pay. If you are self-employed or not currently employed but eligible for a maternity allowance you will need to fill in a claim form (MA1 form), available from your Jobcentre Plus. You will also need a MAT B1 form from your doctor or

PATERNITY LEAVE AND PAY

To qualify for paternity leave and pay you must have been working for a company for 26 weeks or more by the 15th week before the baby is due, and earning over a certain threshold. Paternity leave and pay is available for married and unmarried partners (that is, the biological father), same-sex partners and adoptive fathers. Generally, paternity leave lasts for two weeks, during which statutory paternity pay (SPP) is paid. It usually has to be taken all in one block, within eight weeks of the birth. Some fathers may be entitled to more generous paternity leave and pay, depending on their contract.

midwife to prove your estimated due date and proof of your earnings, such as your payslips.

Free prescriptions and more

During your pregnancy and for a year after the birth of your baby you will be entitled to free prescriptions, NHS dentistry and optical care. Your GP or midwife should fill in a form, which you will also have to sign and send off to the relevant agency. You will then be sent a card that you have to show to obtain free prescriptions.

The Healthy Start Scheme is available in certain cases, such as for women receiving income support. The scheme entitles pregnant women and children under four years old to vouchers that can be used to buy fruit and vegetables, milk or formula milk. If you are eligible for the scheme you will also be entitled to free Healthy Start vitamins during and for one year after your pregnancy. For more information please ask your doctor, midwife or health visitor.

Child benefit, tax credits and parental leave

Once your baby is born, you will be entitled to child benefit, irrespective of your earnings. Depending on your earnings, you may also be entitled to child tax credit or working tax credit. If you have been working for a company for over a year you will be able to take up to 13 weeks of unpaid parental leave until your child is five years old. This leave is for emergency situations, such as looking after a child when they are unwell.

Returning to work

You do not need to give notice of the date of your return to work as your employer must assume you are taking your full year of maternity leave (both paid and unpaid). If you want to return earlier then you must give written notice, at least eight weeks before your intended return to work date.

If you decide that you want to go back to work part-time, then by law your employer has to consider your request. However, this does not mean you will always be able to work flexibly, just that your employer has to make a reasonable effort to accommodate your request. Your partner could also ask to work flexibly, and as long as your child is under six years old his request would also have to be considered.

If you decide not to return to work you should resign as per the conditions in your contract. If you do not have a contract only one week's notice needs to be given. Any notice required can be taken as part of your maternity leave. If you have been given more maternity pay than is statutory as per your contract, you may be required to pay some of it back if you decide not to return to work.

PLANNING AHEAD

It seems complicated – and a long way in the future – but it is important to start thinking about when you would like to stop working, and when you may wish to start working again after your baby is born. This gives you an opportunity to discuss your plans with your boss, although you are still entitled to change your mind. Talking things over with your employer early means that plans can be made regarding your job and maternity cover.

'I was very confused about what I was and wasn't entitled to, and the thought of deciding how much maternity leave to take when I hadn't even had my baby was daunting. I asked for a meeting with my boss and was surprised by how understanding he was. He automatically assumed I would take the whole year, so if I returned earlier it was a bonus for him! We agreed that as long as I gave everyone plenty of notice about when I wanted to go and come back then it would be fine. I am also going to be involved in interviewing a temp for when I'm away, so they really are keeping me in the loop.' Tania, 29

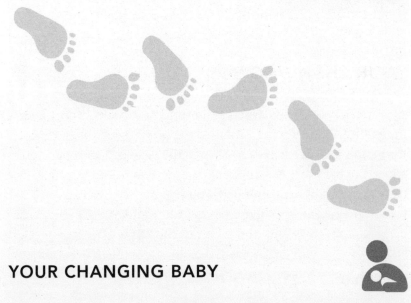

week 22

YOUR CHANGING BABY

By now your baby has a definite sleep–wake cycle, with periods of being active and awake and periods of sleep and rest. You may have already felt some movements, and with time you will be able to differentiate between your baby being asleep and awake by feeling his movements. If he is asleep he can be woken up by your movements or by loud noises, and soon you may feel him jump or startle as he responds to loud noises.

Up until about this point his spleen and liver have been making his blood cells but now his bone marrow (the inside of his long bones) is developed enough to take over this role. His eyes are developing, though as yet he does not have any pigment in his irises (the coloured part of the eye). The hair on his head, eyebrows and eyelashes continues to grow and his skin is still thin and translucent, and pinky red in colour.

If you could see inside the womb, he would look thin and wrinkled, but he is continuing to lay down fat underneath his skin so he will look less wrinkly when he is born. Nipples develop in both boys and girls and he looks like a tiny version of a newborn baby. The amount of weight he puts on each week is increasing. He measures approximately 27.5–28 centimetres (11 inches) in length and weighs about 430 grams (15 ounces).

YOUR CHANGING BODY

At 22 weeks your uterus will measure approximately 22 centimetres in height from its top (the fundus) to your pubic bone. Pregnancy hormones such as relaxin act to soften the ligaments in your pelvis to allow your baby to travel through it during labour. The weight of your baby pushes down on your pelvis and changes your centre of gravity. To compensate for these changes, you walk with a slightly wider gait, leaning backwards and arching your back, giving the typical appearance of a pregnant woman. This loosening of the ligaments combined with the change in posture can result in lower backache during pregnancy. (For more information about how to prevent and relieve backache, see Weeks 24, 27 and 35.)

INDIGESTION AND REFLUX

Indigestion (dyspepsia) and gastro-oesophageal reflux (reflux or heartburn) are extremely common in the later stages of pregnancy. As your uterus expands to accommodate your growing baby there is less room in your abdomen for the rest of your organs. Your stomach is literally squashed by your womb so it has less capacity to hold food. This is why you may need to eat little and often late in pregnancy. High levels of the hormone progesterone relax the muscles in your intestines, making your digestive system slow down so food stays in your stomach for longer. The combination of your relatively small stomach and slower digestive system means that you may get indigestion – a feeling of discomfort in your stomach or upper abdomen. This discomfort can even be sharp pain, and you may feel nauseous.

Reflux or heartburn is also due to the effects of your hormones and physiological changes taking place to accommodate your pregnancy. There is a sphincter between the top of your stomach and the bottom of your oesophagus, which stops food and stomach juices and acids going back up your oesophagus. In pregnancy this sphincter can become relaxed so food and stomach juices and acids can be regurgitated back up, irritating your oesophagus and resulting in a burning pain in your chest.

You may notice that these symptoms improve or even resolve in the very late stages of your pregnancy. This is because as your baby drops and engages into the pelvis, there is more room in your abdomen for your digestive system.

Both indigestion and heartburn should be short lasting and can be relieved with changes to your diet (see opposite) or medication. Medications include Gaviscon, which is safe in pregnancy and available on prescription or over the counter. If you do buy indigestion or heartburn remedies over the counter always inform your pharmacist that you are pregnant as some remedies may not be suitable in pregnancy.

If these remedies are not effective, your doctor may prescribe a medication such as ranitidine, which acts to decrease acid production in your stomach and therefore reduce your symptoms. If you have severe pain and are concerned that it is not indigestion then see your doctor.

'I'd never had indigestion before and the first time I honestly thought I might be having a heart attack. Who knew that it could hurt so much? And I was burping and burping! If I eat too much it sets it off, and I can't eat just before lying down. For me, taking Gaviscon really works – thankfully – so I can keep enjoying my food without worrying about indigestion afterwards!'
Anya, 35

Relieving and preventing indigestion and reflux

Changing your diet and the way that you eat may help relieve symptoms of indigestion and reflux. Firstly, eat sitting upright and not lounging against cushions on your sofa; sitting upright may create more space in your abdomen, relieving some of the compressing forces on your stomach. After you have eaten, try to avoid lying down for at least an hour, allowing gravity to help keep the food in your stomach to prevent reflux. Avoid eating in the few hours before going to bed. If you have eaten prior to going to sleep, try propping yourself up on several pillows to keep your head up, as if you are half sitting up, again to allow gravity to help prevent reflux.

Consider keeping a food diary. This involves writing down what you eat and whether or not you then had any symptoms. You may find that certain foods trigger indigestion, commonly very spicy or fatty foods or foods that are very acidic, such as pickled items or citrus fruits. Other triggers include caffeine, alcohol and smoking, although hopefully you are limiting your caffeine and alcohol intake and are not smoking. Avoiding large heavy meals and eating little and often may relieve your symptoms. The traditional remedy of drinking a glass of milk before eating or going to bed may also help to neutralise any acid (as milk is alkaline), and natural yoghurt may work in a similar way. Some people find ginger or peppermint tea helps settle their tummy.

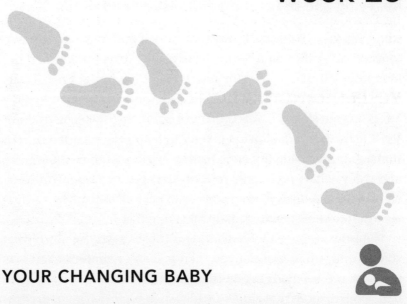

week 23

YOUR CHANGING BABY

Although your baby's head and body are more in proportion than previously, he still has a large head and will have a proportionally big head even when he is born. His lips have developed and, if you were to have a scan at this stage, you might be able to see him sucking his thumb. His tongue is formed and his taste buds are developed enough to differentiate between salty, sweet and bitter tastes, though he isn't eating anything yet. The tooth buds in his gums are forming; these will eventually develop into his milk teeth, which won't be seen for at least a few months after birth.

He continues to practise moving, getting his exercise by kicking, moving from side to side and turning over. There is still enough room in your womb for lots of movement, and he can even turn somersaults. The bones and nerves of his inner ear have developed; the inner ear is involved with balance, so he may even be able to tell if he is upside down!

His intestines continue to mature and his pancreas can produce insulin, which is involved in the control of blood sugar levels. He continues to lay down fat and put on weight, though he still looks very thin. His skin starts to lay down pigment, changing from almost see-through and pinkish to the skin colour he will be born with. He measures approximately 28–29 centimetres (11–11½ inches) and weighs about 500 grams (1 pound 2 ounces).

YOUR CHANGING BODY

In order to accommodate your expanding uterus, which in turn is making room for your growing baby, other organs in your abdomen and chest undergo changes. Your ribs move upwards and the lower ribs also spread sideways to create more space below; this means that there is less room in your chest to take deep breaths so you may begin to feel breathless. Your stomach and intestines move up into this space and spread either side of your growing womb. There is less room than previously so your digestive tract becomes squashed. As your womb grows and all these changes occur, you may get the occasional ache or stretching-type pain in your abdomen. If any pain is severe or constant, however, see your doctor.

URINARY TRACT INFECTIONS

Women are more prone than men to developing urinary tract infections due to the relatively short length of the female urethra – the tube that carries urine from your bladder to the outside. This means that any bacteria have only a short distance to travel before they can infect your bladder. The high levels of progesterone in your body during pregnancy relax the structures of your urinary tract (kidneys, bladder and the connecting tubing), making it even easier for bacteria to travel up into the bladder to cause an infection. The relaxation also means that if you do have a bladder infection (cystitis) it is easier for the bacteria to travel further up into the kidneys, causing a kidney infection (pyelonephritis). It is important to treat urinary tract infections. If untreated they can cause long-term kidney problems, and in later pregnancy can irritate the uterus and cause contractions.

Symptoms of urinary tract infections include urinary frequency – going to the toilet to pass urine more than usual. Urinary frequency alone is extremely common in pregnancy. However, if you find that you are going to the toilet even more often than you have come to expect to be normal in your pregnancy, you may have an infection. Other symptoms include lower abdominal pain or aching, and a painful burning or stinging sensation as you pass urine. If the kidneys are also involved you may develop a high fever with shaking and shivering, and abdominal or back pain which may radiate downwards into your groin.

If you have any of these symptoms see your doctor who will prescribe appropriate antibiotics. Your doctor may also send off a sample of your urine to the lab to check that the bacteria are sensitive to the antibiotics used. It is important that you finish the course of antibiotics, even if you are feeling better, to prevent the bacteria developing resistance to antibiotics.

If you have a urine sample sent to the lab for another reason, such as for protein in the urine, a urine infection is sometimes found, even though you may not have any symptoms. This is called asymptomatic bacteriuria and still needs treatment with antibiotics to prevent complications which can lead to kidney infections and premature labour.

FOR FATHERS

During the second trimester you will hopefully notice that your partner is feeling better physically and probably has more energy than in the earlier stages of pregnancy. She will become aware of the baby moving inside her, and in a little while you will be able to feel him kicking through her tummy. You might like to spend time with your partner, talking about the baby and your hopes and any anxieties about parenthood. You could stroke your partner's bump and talk or sing to it, to help feel connected to your developing baby.

'It was strange. After weeks of vomiting she suddenly went back to normal; in fact, better than normal. She had loads of energy and started planning lots of jobs for me, like building a cot! I remember feeling left out when she started feeling the movements. She would suddenly go all quiet and still, like she was turning in on herself, and say that she felt something. I couldn't be a part of that so when I could feel the kicks it was amazing. Then I had my hands on the bump all the time, waiting to feel my baby kick – I was convinced I had a star striker in the making.' Simon, 38

YOGA

Seated poses are thought to be good to help open the hips and groin, and keep the muscles in these areas flexible. You may like to try the following poses:

Staff pose

This is often the starting position for other seated poses. Sit on the floor with your legs out in front of you. You may wish to put a folded towel under your bottom for support. Engage the muscles in your thighs, squeezing them together, and flex your feet upwards so your heels may come off the floor. Sit up straight, thinking about extending your spine with each vertebra directly on top of the one below, keeping your head straight as you look ahead. Breathe.

Cobbler's pose

This helps open the hips. You may find sitting on a small cushion or folded towel helpful to open the hips. Start in the staff pose, then bend your knees and place the soles of your feet together, so that your legs make a diamond shape. Press your soles together and let your knees fall apart; you may wish to put towels under your knees to support them. Sit tall, keeping your spine long and stretched if you can. Hold on to your feet with your hands and remember to keep breathing.

'She looks amazing, kind of glowing and so happy. And her body is fantastic, all soft and curvy with a lovely rounded bump that has my baby in it. What could be more feminine and sexy than that?' Martin, 32

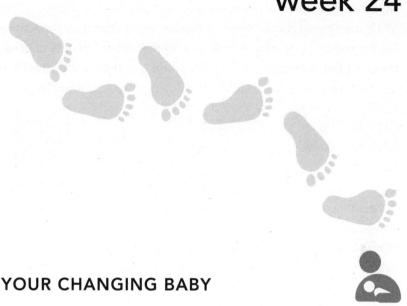

week 24

YOUR CHANGING BABY

Your baby continues to put on weight, now about 90–100 grams (3–3½ ounces) per week. This weight gain is made up of his muscles, bones and body fat, which will help keep him warm and give him energy once he is born.

His lungs continue to mature and begin to produce a substance called surfactant. This acts to keep the tiny air sacs in the lungs, called alveoli, open; to expand them on his first breath and then prevent them from collapsing, thus helping him breathe. He practises the movements of breathing, moving his chest up and down as he inhales and exhales amniotic fluid.

His hands develop creases in the palms, and soon sweat glands will form in his skin. He measures approximately 30 centimetres (11¾ inches) in length and weighs about 600 grams (1 pound 5 ounces).

YOUR CHANGING BODY

By Week 24 of your pregnancy, if you are carrying a single baby your uterus measures approximately 24 centimetres (9½ inches) from its fundus to your pubic bone. Hopefully your bump will not be too large yet so you should still be comfortable and unhindered by it. Despite the many changes going on, both in your body and that of your baby, many women report feeling fantastic during the second trimester.

CHANGING POSTURE AND BACK PAIN

As your bump increases in size you will have more weight than usual in the front middle section of your body. This extra weight changes your centre of gravity. If you don't adjust how you stand and walk, it could make you topple over forwards. In order to stop this, women walk and stand with their legs further apart than before pregnancy. This wider stance helps you feel more balanced and happens subconsciously. Women also notice that they lean back, arching their lower back to compensate for the weight of their bump.

The high levels of pregnancy hormones such as relaxin mean that the connective tissues in the ligaments of your pelvis (the tissues that connect bones) have relaxed. This relaxation allows the pelvis to expand to accommodate the baby and enable it to come out through the birth canal during labour. The increasing weight of your bump puts further pressure on your pelvis. These factors combine to make your pelvis less stable than prior to pregnancy. The positions you adopt to counteract your changing centre of gravity can often lead to backache as the connective tissues in the pelvis can become strained. Back pain is extremely common in pregnancy, so try to avoid putting on more weight than is expected for pregnancy (for more information see page 65) as it will put more pressure on your back.

How to prevent back pain

Making some adjustments to your posture, your shoes and how you move may prevent some back pain, or at least stop any discomfort from getting worse.

- You may find that lying on your side relieves the pressure on your lower back. (For information about how to get up from lying down safely with a bump see page 211.)
- Try to ensure that you sit straight with some support for your lower back, either from the back of the chair or a cushion.
- If you are sitting for long periods, such as at work, make sure that your chair is comfortable and the correct height for you. You should be able to place both feet flat on the floor comfortably, to rest your arms on the desk in front of you without having to lift them up and to look straight ahead at a computer screen without having to look or tilt your face upwards.
- Try to stand as straight as you can. Avoid slouching forward over your bump, and try not to overarch the small of your back.
- As your pregnancy continues, you will probably find that wearing high-heeled shoes becomes more uncomfortable. This is because your feet may have become slightly swollen due to the increased fluid in your body, but also because high heels further exaggerate the postural changes you are already making to compensate for your bump. When wearing high heels you may find that you have to arch your back even further to compensate for the increased instability, which can make any back discomfort worse. Shoes with low heels, or flat shoes with some support for the arches of your feet, will probably be more comfortable.
- Try to avoid lifting heavy weights, but if you do have to – such as when picking up another child – bend your knees and squat down before lifting. As you pick up your child (or other heavy object) push up with the strong muscles in your legs and try to keep your back straight.
- Doing some back exercises, such as the pelvic tilts described in Week 25, yoga, Pilates or swimming can help strengthen the muscles in your back.
- If you do get some discomfort, a relaxing back rub can be helpful. Ask your partner or treat yourself to a pregnancy massage.
- As your pregnancy progresses and your bump gets larger, you may find that a support belt helps relieve some of the strain. These can

be bought from most parenting and baby stores such as Mother-care, or may be available from a physiotherapist.

A LEGAL MILESTONE

Currently, the legal definition of viability in the UK is 24 weeks' gestation. Babies born before 24 weeks who show no signs of life do not have to be registered and are classified as a miscarriage. After 24 weeks the chance of survival steadily begins to increase. However, the earlier a baby is born the more likely it is to need resuscitation and intense medical care and have long-term disabilities. The longer the time spent in the womb, the more time the baby has to develop and mature. If your baby is born early you will be able to start your maternity leave from the date of delivery.

Passing the 24th week is often an emotional milestone. From now on many women feel that the pregnancy is real, and that the baby is really coming!

'It feels like I am now entering a new stage, and with every day that passes the baby becomes almost more alive to me.' Yvette, 41

week 25

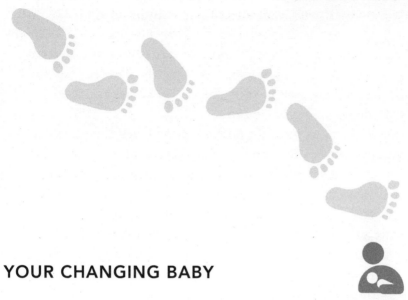

YOUR CHANGING BABY

Your baby continues to mature: his brain is getting bigger and the brain cells are still developing. He has the ability to respond to all of his senses. More complex cells, whose function is to do with consciousness, memory, perception and the ability to learn, also develop. If you measure his brainwaves, they are similar to those of a newborn baby.

The many tiny bones of the spine begin to form. His hands are developed and his dexterity is improving all the time. He can grasp things in his fist and even play with his umbilical cord by pulling on it. He sucks his thumb and plays with his hands and feet, learning by moving, touching and exploring. His face continues to develop with his nostrils opening, though they will be filled with amniotic fluid. He measures approximately 34 centimetres (1 foot 1 inch) and weighs about 660–690 grams (1 pound 8 ounces).

YOUR CHANGING BODY

Your peripheral blood vessels continue to dilate to stop your blood pressure rising as your blood volume and cardiac output keep increasing. The increased blood supply to your skin, along with high levels of oestrogen, can affect the condition of your skin. These changes often lead to soft skin and rosy cheeks, described as the 'glow of pregnancy'. Not all women notice this change, however; in some, the high hormone levels may make the skin dry or spotty. The dilated blood vessels in your skin can sometimes be seen, so your skin may look pink or blotchy.

Your hair may also look different during pregnancy, again due to the effect of your hormones, becoming very thick and glossy. This is because your hair is growing faster than normal and less is falling out. Hair all over your body, not just on your head, grows faster during pregnancy. After the baby is born you will notice that you are losing more hair than normal, or even that your hair is becoming quite thin in comparison to how it was during pregnancy. Don't worry: this is just the hair that would have normally fallen out over the last nine months all coming out over a much shorter time so it looks like a lot! You may also notice that your nails grow faster during pregnancy; again, this is due to the effects of your hormones.

Constipation

High levels of the hormone progesterone make the muscles in your intestines relax, slowing down your digestive system. This means that you are more likely to develop constipation during pregnancy. Constipation is when you are going to the toilet to open your bowels less regularly than is normal for you and the stool is hard and difficult to pass. It can also make you feel bloated or give you abdominal pain.

To try to prevent or treat constipation look at your diet: increase the amount of fluid that you drink and eat lots of fruit, vegetables and whole grains to increase the amount of fibre in your diet. This should help keep your stool soft and easy to pass. Exercising can also help prevent or relieve constipation. If these simple measures do not work, then over-the-counter laxatives such as Fybogel are safe in pregnancy. When buying over-the-counter remedies, be sure to inform your pharmacist that you are pregnant so they can check that the remedy you are buying is appropriate for use in pregnancy. Fybogel is a bulking agent, which causes you to absorb more water into your stool to make it soft. If these do not work then visit your doctor who will be able to prescribe a stronger medication such as lactulose.

ANTENATAL APPOINTMENT

If this is your first baby you will be offered an antenatal appointment at around the 25th week of your pregnancy. Your blood pressure will be taken, your urine will be tested and you will be examined. If you are having any concerns, be sure to discuss them with your doctor or midwife at this appointment.

PLANNING AHEAD: CHILDCARE OPTIONS

At this stage you might like to start thinking and planning ahead regarding childcare if you decide to return to work. Many childcare providers may get booked up months in advance. Options include:

- Your partner staying at home.
- Asking relatives, such as your parents, to help out. It is important to take into consideration their opinions regarding raising children. For example, if your parents would want your child to be in a strict routine, but you don't, it could cause tension. Just as you would for a childminder or nanny, discuss the kind of care you want for your child with your relatives, so you are all in agreement!

- A registered childminder who looks after a few children in their own home.
- A nursery, either private or state run. These have varying hours of work.
- A nanny. This is probably the most expensive option. Here your child will have one-to-one care with a registered and qualified nanny. Nannies can be both live-in, where they live in your home, or live-out.
- An au-pair. This is generally a young person – often not from the UK – who lives in your house and looks after your child. They may also do some domestic jobs. They may not have any previous childcare experience.

Each of these options has its advantages and disadvantages. You can obtain a list of local childminders and nurseries from your local council.

'People keep asking me what I am going to do with the baby when I go back to work. I only went on maternity leave three days ago and everyone asks when I am going back – I don't know! I realise I have to plan ahead but I haven't even met the baby yet. How can I interview a childminder?' Stacey, 28

ANTENATAL CLASSES

You may have booked a place on an antenatal class earlier in your pregnancy, generally through your hospital, local branch of the National Childbirth Trust or a private midwife. Women tend to start attending classes towards the end of the second trimester. Classes can be in the daytime, evening or at weekends, depending on your

'I was really nervous about starting antenatal classes and almost had to physically drag my husband along, but I am glad that I went. Not only was it an opportunity to ask some of the many questions I had, but it was also a chance to meet other pregnant women. I am the first of my friends to get pregnant so it was great to slowly make friends with other people who understood what I was going through, and were happy to let me talk about being pregnant, and afterwards my baby, all the time!' Phoebe, 26

particular course. You are entitled to time off to attend them, though your employer may ask for a certificate of attendance to prove that you went to the class.

The classes are aimed at both men and women. They are not simply about breathing techniques, but about giving you information so that you can both make informed choices. Classes will cover various topics including common complaints during pregnancy, signs of labour, labour itself and the various options for pain relief. There will also be discussions about life after the birth, breastfeeding, changing nappies and bathing. Perhaps most importantly, classes are an opportunity to meet other women or couples in similar circumstances to your own, so that you can share your woes and joys together!

YOGA: PELVIC TILTS

These can be performed lying down or standing up
and are great for the pelvis and lower back, and may
help relieve any lower back or pelvic discomfort.
Standing may be more comfortable in later
pregnancy when you should not lie flat on your back.
Stand with your back against a wall, with your feet
and legs slightly in front. Your feet should be a little
more than hip-width apart and your knees slightly
bent. Exhale while you tilt your pelvis upwards. As
you do this you should feel your back press against
the wall. Inhale as you return to the start position
and repeat.

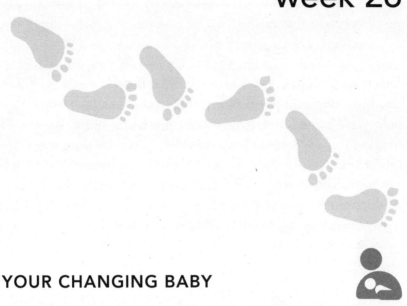

week 26

YOUR CHANGING BABY

Your baby's brain continues to mature, and brainwaves can be measured from different parts of the brain. He is moving a lot; during the late second trimester and beginning of the third trimester, he still has proportionally lots of room to move around. As time progresses he will get bigger in relation to your womb and will have less room to move. When he kicks, your partner may be able to feel it through your tummy. He may repeat actions that he enjoys; sucking his thumb, for instance, helps to strengthen the muscles in his face and jaw so that he can suck well to get milk after he is born.

You now have about 500 millilitres (17½ fluid ounces) of amniotic fluid, which is recycled as your baby swallows and urinates. He measures approximately 35.5 centimetres (1 foot 2 inches) and weighs about 760 grams (1 pound 10 ounces).

YOUR CHANGING BODY

By Week 26 of your pregnancy, your womb will be about 26 centimetres (10 inches) in height. Your blood volume continues to rise, to about 5 litres (8¾ pints), and consequently your heart will beat out more blood per heartbeat.

The changes of pregnancy can also affect your mind. You might find yourself having strange dreams, not necessarily about your pregnancy or baby, and many women find that they become forgetful or clumsy during their pregnancy. This is sometimes called 'pregnancy brain' and can be quite frustrating! You might become forgetful because you are focused on your baby, or on any symptoms you might be having; or it may be related to your pregnancy hormones. Whatever the cause, women find that their forgetfulness often persists during the first few weeks or even months after their baby is born, when sleep deprivation may also be a factor.

Dizziness

Some women may have felt dizzy during the first trimester. Others may have just noticed that they occasionally feel dizzy, especially when getting up from lying down, or if they have been standing for long periods. The reasons behind feeling dizzy are described in Week 13.

To try to prevent dizziness, make sure that you get up slowly from lying or sitting down to allow your body to compensate. If you are standing for long periods, keep moving your legs to help the blood be pumped back to the heart and stop it pooling in your lower limbs. If you do feel dizzy, sit down, open your legs and put your head between your knees (letting your bump fall between your legs), or lie down with your feet up – this makes it easier for the heart to pump blood to the brain as it does not have to work against gravity. Low blood sugar levels can also make you feel dizzy so make sure you are eating regularly.

'I'm so tired!'

You may have also noticed that you are beginning to feel tired, even if you are well rested. This is unsurprising. Your body is undergoing major changes under the influence of your pregnancy hormones;

you are carrying around extra weight and your metabolic rate has increased. Put simply, your body is working much harder than it used to, so you feel tired.

Try to rest as much as you can, perhaps taking short naps in the day if possible. If you are working then you could try talking to your boss; there may be some work you could do from home, or you could change your working hours slightly so you don't travel in the crowded rush hour. Even making sure that you have enough time to eat properly, or have a drink and a sit down for five minutes, can help. Delegate and share your responsibilities, and remember that this can apply both at work and at home, such as to the housework. Listen to your body – it will tell you when you've had enough!

PRE-ECLAMPSIA

During pregnancy, your blood pressure normally falls as your blood vessels relax and dilate to cope with the extra blood volume flowing through them. If you have high blood pressure before your pregnancy, or are diagnosed with high blood pressure at less than 20 weeks' pregnancy, you will probably be referred to a hospital obstetrician. They will check and, if appropriate, change your antihypertensive (high blood pressure) medication.

About 5–10 per cent of pregnancies are complicated by the development of pregnancy-induced hypertension – high blood pressure in pregnancy. The majority of cases occur in first pregnancies, in the second half of pregnancy, and are mild. Approximately 2–5 per cent of pregnancies are complicated by pre-eclampsia. In this condition, the blood pressure also rises but, unlike in pregnancy-induced hypertension, other systems of the body are affected. You may, for example, have protein in your urine.

It is not known exactly what causes pre-eclampsia or how it can be prevented but it is important to attend your antenatal appointments so you can be monitored for signs of the condition. At every antenatal visit you will be asked about the symptoms of pre-eclampsia, which are swelling of the feet, ankles, legs and hands, and even the face; headache, and any visual problems. Your blood pressure will also be measured and your urine checked for the presence of protein. It is difficult to give an exact figure of what high blood pressure in pregnancy is as it may depend on what your readings were during the early stages of your pregnancy. In general, blood pressure above 150/100 will need treatment.

Pre-eclampsia can cause problems with pregnancy. If it is severe, blood flow to the placenta may be reduced so the baby may not grow properly. If you do develop pre-eclampsia you will have regular ultrasound scans to check how things are going. The treatment of pre-eclampsia will depend on how high your blood pressure is and how far along in your pregnancy you are, and generally involves oral medication to bring down the blood pressure. Pregnancy-induced hypertension is effectively cured by delivering the baby, but a balance needs to be weighed up between delivering a baby early, with the risks that involves, and the risks to both the baby and the mother of continuing.

If the blood pressure rises suddenly, or becomes very high, there is a risk of eclampsia developing. This is a serious condition in which seizures and even coma can occur. It is treated with various medications and immediate delivery, usually by Caesarean section. As with many topics in medicine, this does sound frightening; however, remember that you will be closely monitored and treated with medication to try and prevent this happening.

DIET

You may have noticed that you are unable to eat three full meals a day as your stomach has shrunk due to your growing uterus. This means that you feel full quicker and need to eat little and often. Do not skip breakfast as this will increase the likelihood of you developing low blood sugar levels and feeling faint. Even if this doesn't happen, skipping breakfast can make you feel tired, sluggish and irritable, and more likely to snack on unhealthy foods later on in the morning when you get hungry. If you can't face breakfast then try drinking a fresh smoothie – one made with fruit for example – or eating a yoghurt and oat flakes to help get you going.

If you need to snack regularly then try to avoid fatty, high-sugar snacks. These will bring your blood sugar levels up rapidly but they will soon fall and may leave you feeling worse and hungrier than before. Carry some healthy snacks such as dried fruit, nuts, rice cakes or cereal bars so that you have something available if you need to eat.

> 'I'm like a walking shop. I have stashes of food everywhere – in my handbag, in my car, in my desk at work, everywhere! I find if I eat big meals I get indigestion so I graze, eating lots of little things – various bags of nuts and seeds, fruit and of course the occasional and essential chocolate!' Priya, 39

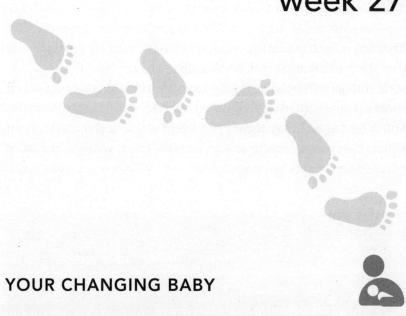

week 27

YOUR CHANGING BABY

Your baby's irises will have started to develop their pigment. If his eyes were open you would be able to see what colour they are, though the colour may change after birth. He can open and close his eyes and responds to light and dark – if you shine a light on your tummy he can respond by turning away from it. He still can't see very well, though, as he has a short focal length, which means he is short-sighted. He will still be short-sighted when he is born but will be able to see the distance between your breast and your face so you can look at each other while you are breastfeeding, perfect for bonding.

His lungs continue to develop and produce surfactant, a substance that helps keep the air sacs from collapsing when he starts to breathe, and he is still practising the all-important movements for breathing. His brain is still growing, and begins to take on its characteristic grooved appearance. His immune system begins to develop, helped by your antibodies that can cross the placenta. He measures approximately 36.5 centimetres (1 foot 2½ inches) in length and weighs about 875 grams (1 pound 15 ounces).

YOUR CHANGING BODY

Your ribs continue to rise and spread outwards to create more space in your abdominal cavity for your expanding uterus. This can cause some discomfort around the ribcage, especially if your baby is breech (head up instead of head down into your pelvis) and bumps your ribs. You might notice these changes more when you are sitting down when there is even less space in your abdomen, so try standing or lying down to relieve any discomfort.

'By the time I get to the top of the stairs, I'm completely out of puff!'

As the second trimester ends you may notice that you feel breathless or that you become short of breath much more easily than normal. This is because your expanding womb is pushing up against your diaphragm, the large muscle at the base of your lungs. The diaphragm cannot fully flatten during an inhalation, so you can't take as big a breath as previously. Again, due to your expanding bump, your lower ribs have moved sideways, flaring outwards. Your diaphragm connects to these lower ribs, and as they move outwards they stretch the diaphragm so it becomes less elastic than normal and cannot move as much, again reducing the amount you can inhale.

As well as these mechanical pressures, the hormone progesterone makes you breathe faster than normal to ensure you receive enough oxygen. The combination of these factors can make you feel breathless, or have the sensation that you are hyperventilating. Sometimes this can also make you feel dizzy.

FAMILY AND FRIENDS

Many women report that their relationships change during their pregnancy. Being pregnant and having a child, be it a first or subsequent baby, affects all areas of your life, including the relationships you have with friends and family. You may find that you feel closer to your mother or other women who have had children, who can empathise with your experiences. Your relationship with your partner may be changing. If this is your first baby the focus moves from just the two of you to being a threesome; or if this is a second or third child, to your expanding family. You and your partner may have concerns about money. He may suddenly become the sole breadwinner for the family, with new responsibilities and concerns.

Relationships with friends may also change. You may find distance developing between yourself and friends without babies, as your priorities in life are currently very different. These changes can be difficult, but try to remember that relationships are always changing and fluctuating. Talk to your friends and family and let them explain to you how they are feeling. Allowing each other the time to talk and, perhaps even more importantly, to listen will hopefully

Some women worry that they will not be able to love or pay attention to everyone, but the capacity of a mother to love her children is endless and there is always enough to go round.

'Already our relationship has gone from being just the two of us, to being about the three of us. We already take the baby into consideration and are planning for the future and it hasn't even arrived yet!' Adelaide, 31

keep your friendships close; or, if not, will allow them to become more distant without animosity.

MANAGING BACK PAIN

As mentioned earlier, back pain is extremely common in pregnancy. However, if you are concerned, or if the pain is severe and limits your activities, do ask your doctor to examine you to check that it is nothing more serious. Try to prevent back pain developing by protecting your back using the methods described in Week 24. A support belt or maternity belt may help relieve some of your symptoms. These belts are worn just underneath your bump, supporting some of the weight on your pelvis. They can be worn during the day but should be removed at night.

If back pain is bothering you then there are painkillers that are safe in pregnancy, such as paracetamol (for more information see page 19). Your doctor will be able to prescribe you further pain medication if paracetamol is not sufficient. They may also be able to refer you to a women's health or maternity physiotherapist who may be able to give you further exercises and massage to relieve your discomfort.

> 'My job involves me being on my feet all day, every day, and by the middle of my pregnancy I was really feeling it in my lower back. I spoke to my boss and was able to change what I did a little bit so I had some time sitting down. I was also referred to a physio who really helped.' Stacey, 30

Doing exercises, such as those described overleaf, to strengthen the muscles of your lower back and pelvis and improve your posture will be helpful. Exercise also releases endorphins, the body's feel-good chemicals, which can act to relieve pain or at least make you feel a little better. Do not continue any exercise if it is causing discomfort.

- Lie on the floor on your back and gently hug your knees (you will need to open your knees slightly to accommodate your bump). Relax then rock gently from side to side to stretch the lower back. This exercise also massages the lower spine as you rock from side to side.
- Still on your back, bend your knees and lift your feet into the air, feet together, so that your hips and knees are at right angles. Then twist to drop your knees to one side as you turn your head in the opposite direction. Repeat on the other side, gently stretching the spine.
- Get on your hands and knees (on all fours) and then try to gently move your right hip towards your right shoulder. Return to the centre before moving your left hip to your left shoulder, rather as if you were a dog wagging its tail.

Yoga positions such as pelvic tilts (see Week 25), child's pose (see Week 28) and cat-cow sequence (see Week 36) help to stretch and strengthen the spine.

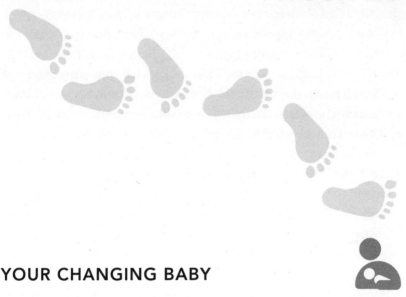

week 28

YOUR CHANGING BABY

Your baby's nostrils and lungs are filled with amniotic fluid. This is generally squeezed out as he passes through the birth canal during labour; Caesarean babies may sneeze it out once they are born. The lungs are not yet fully mature and continue to develop. Tiny air sacs called alveoli form, which continue to form after he is born. If he is born before about 34 or 35 weeks' gestation, not enough alveoli will have developed, and there may not be enough surfactant – the substance that helps him breathe. As a result, his lungs would be stiff and he might need help with breathing.

His nervous system matures further as sheaths of myelin are laid down around nerves to speed up the electrical transmission of nerve impulses. He continues to move around and may spend more time in positions he finds comfortable, such as the 'foetal position' with his arms and legs pulled into his chest. His eyelids are open and his eyes can move around to look from side to side. During his sleep, rapid eye movement (REM) brainwaves can be seen, which may mean that your baby is dreaming.

Keep talking to your baby. You will find that your voice can calm him. Studies have shown that, even in the womb, a baby's heart rate can drop in response to his mother's voice. Your baby may now have developed enough for you to play with him. At a time when you know he is awake and active, try tapping on your bump – he can feel it when you touch your bump and may give a kick in response. You can then tap back. As you tap and he kicks you are communicating with each other! He may also respond when you massage your bump. Encourage your partner to talk to your baby too, so that he will recognise both your voices after birth.

By this point in pregnancy there can be significant variation in weight and length of babies, due to genetic, nutritional and other differences. How big your baby will be will depend on, among other things, the size of you and your partner; whether you smoke or are diabetic; whether you are carrying a multiple pregnancy. The average foetus at this stage measures approximately 37.5 centimetres (1 foot 2¾ inches) in length and weighs about 1 kilogram (2 pounds 3 ounces).

YOUR CHANGING BODY

There is now less room round the sides of your uterus and so your digestive system is displaced upwards and squashed. You may notice that you have to eat little and often as your stomach can hold less food than normal. Although your baby, placenta and womb will continue to grow, from approximately 36 weeks the head may become engaged (though this can be later if this isn't your first pregnancy). This means the baby drops lower into the pelvis, leaving a bit more room in your tummy and relieving some of the pressure.

Haemorrhoids

Haemorrhoids, or piles, are a common complaint during pregnancy. There is a network of veins in and around your anus. If these veins become dilated they are called haemorrhoids. These dilated veins can then become thrombosed, which means they are full of clotted blood. All the blood vessels in the body are relaxed during pregnancy. Haemorrhoids form because the weight of your bump pushing down into your pelvis prevents the blood in your veins from travelling back to your heart, so the veins dilate and expand.

Piles can be itchy and bleed. You tend to notice bright red blood on the toilet paper after you wipe yourself. They can also be painful or throb. You may be able to feel a lump around your back passage, which you may or may not be able to push back into your anus.

Constipation can make haemorrhoids worse as you push and strain when trying to open your bowels, further increasing the pressure. To avoid getting constipated eat lots of fruit and vegetables to boost your fibre intake, and be sure to drink plenty of fluids.

The throbbing sensation, discomfort or itching of piles may be relieved by applying a soothing cold or ice pack to the area or using a haemorrhoid cream such as Anusol. Creams can be bought over the counter (though inform your pharmacist that you are pregnant). They contain a lubricant to make it easier to open your bowels and a local anaesthetic to relieve any pain.

'Every now and again I round up my pregnancy symptoms: constipation – tick, haemorrhoids – tick, heartburn – sometimes, so tick; can't walk upstairs without being short of breath – tick. Then I round up the ones I haven't got – varicose veins, back pain, leg cramps. My pregnant friends and I compare symptoms! But behind it all I know that I would put up with anything. These are all normal parts of pregnancy. There is a baby coming so it's worth it!' Charlotte, 29

ANTENATAL APPOINTMENT

At around 28 weeks your antenatal team will do some routine blood tests. These tests include a full blood count to check that you have not become anaemic and require iron tablets. Your blood type will also be checked again, and if you are Rhesus negative you will be offered an injection of anti-D to prevent you building up antibodies against the baby (for more information see Week 11). In some units you will receive two doses of anti-D – one now at 28 weeks and another at 34 weeks – though other units (using a different dose) give only a single injection at 28 weeks. You will be given a further dose after delivery and if there are complications such as bleeding during the pregnancy, or if you have a procedure during the pregnancy, such as external cephalic version (ECV) – for more information see page 217.

As at every antenatal appointment your blood pressure and urine sample will be checked, the height of your womb will be measured and your midwife or doctor will listen to the baby's heart.

Your baby's position

Your baby is now big enough for your team to determine its position – whether it is lying vertically (longitudinal lie), diagonally (oblique lie) or horizontally (transverse lie). If your baby is lying longitudinally your doctor or midwife will also try to determine its presentation.

The term presentation refers to the part of your baby that is closest to the pelvis. If your baby is head down, the position is called cephalic; head up and bottom or feet down, the position is breech. Don't worry if your doctor cannot tell you the presentation of the baby – it can be difficult to differentiate a head from a bottom at this stage! Babies need to be in the vertical or longitudinal position to deliver, be they cephalic or breech, but don't worry if your baby is not as there is plenty of time and space for him to change position at this point in the pregnancy. If you are carrying twins then either twin can be in any lie or presentation. For example, both babies may be lying vertically with cephalic presentations, or one may be cephalic and the second breech.

EXAMPLES OF LIE

Vertical Transverse Oblique

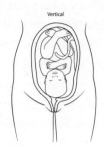 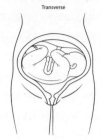 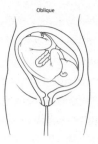

PRESENTATION

Cephalic Complete Breech Frank Breech Footling Breech

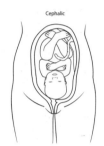 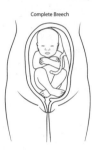 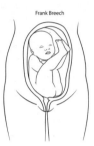 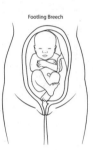

Glucose tolerance test

The glucose tolerance test is a test for gestational diabetes, a condition where you cannot control the levels of sugar in your blood. Gestational diabetes is a relatively common condition of pregnancy and can lead to complications such as the baby having low blood sugar levels after delivery. In some maternity departments you will be offered a test only if you have a first-degree relative (parent or sibling) with diabetes; if you had gestational diabetes in a previous pregnancy; if you previously had a large baby (over 4.5 kilograms/ 9 pounds 15 ounces) or had a high glucose level on a blood test.

The test is generally performed at the end of the second or beginning of the third trimester, generally around 28 weeks, or between 26 and 30 weeks. You will be asked to come in in the morning and to fast from midnight the night before, meaning you should not eat anything and drink only water (not juice or any other fluid). When you get to the hospital you may be asked to give a urine sample, and a fasting baseline blood test will be taken. You will then be given a 'glucose load' – this is generally in the form of a sugary drink, which is often very sweet and can be quite thick. Many women find it quite unpalatable on an empty stomach. Depending on your maternity unit you will then either have a second blood test after two hours, or will have finger-prick blood tests every half an hour for two hours. The tests aim to show how your body deals with glucose (sugar), and whether or not it is able to produce enough insulin, or respond to insulin sufficiently, to prevent your blood sugar levels getting too high.

The results may take a few days to be processed. If there is a problem you will probably be contacted before your next antenatal appointment. If you are found to have gestational diabetes you may be asked to come for extra appointments and scans (for more information see page 172).

YOGA

Both the poses described below can be used for relaxation. Child's pose is also used as a resting pose between other poses. You may find it eases aches and pains in the lower back as it stretches and strengthens the spine. Some people find the hero pose so comfortable that they use it when meditating.

Child's pose

In this pose it is important that you do not put any pressure on your bump. Start off on all fours, then bring your feet together so your lower legs make a V shape and lean back to put your bottom on your heels with your forehead on the floor. In a kneeling position, stretch your arms over your head. Open your knees so that your bump can nestle between your knees. You can use a stack of pillows or blocks to support your head, arms and chest if necessary. Breathe and feel the stretch down your back. To come out of the pose, come up on to all fours before standing up.

Hero pose

This pose helps to stabilise and centre your hips. Start by kneeling with your knees slightly wider than hip width apart. Place a block or rolled blanket or towel between your feet so that as you sit down your bottom lands on it. Sit so your bottom is resting on your support with your belly falling between your knees. Sit up straight, thinking about each bone of your spine being stacked directly on top of the one below. To come out of hero pose you should move on to all fours before standing.

In this position you may wish to add a neck stretch which may help with neck stiffness. Bend your neck as if your right ear is trying to touch your right shoulder, then bring your right hand over to the left side of your head to hold your left ear and help slightly increase the stretch. Drop your left arm straight down to the floor. Breathe then repeat on the other side.

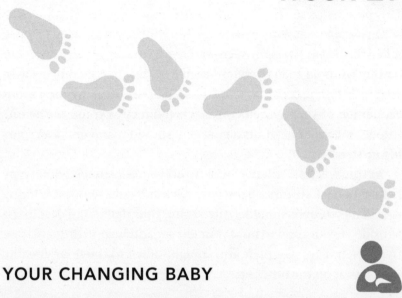

week 29

YOUR CHANGING BABY

By now all your baby's organs have developed and are functioning (apart from the lungs, which are not yet needed to transfer oxygen into the bloodstream). The organs will continue to mature in the coming weeks and months before birth. His head increases in size to accommodate his rapidly growing brain, which has developed enough to let him feel touch and pain. His eyes continue to develop and his pupils can now contract and dilate in response to light, which he can see through the wall of your womb and the increasingly stretched skin of your tummy.

In boys, the testicles begin to move from the abdomen into the groin to end up in the scrotum; in girls, the ovaries are already in the pelvis. The external genitals in girls continue to develop as the labia begin to grow to cover the clitoris. The average foetus measures approximately 38.5 centimetres (1 foot 3 inches) in length and weighs about 1.15 kilograms (2 pounds 8 ounces). In the next weeks and months your baby will continue to grow and put on weight, approximately tripling his current weight.

YOUR CHANGING BODY

By this stage your baby and womb will have grown so much that they will be putting pressure on your bladder. Your bladder no longer has room to expand and therefore hold as much urine as it used to before pregnancy, so you will need to urinate much more frequently. Towards the end of your pregnancy as your baby's head engages into your pelvis, there is even less room for your bladder to expand and you may find yourself going to the toilet even more often! You might also have noticed that you leak small amounts of urine when you laugh, cough or jump. This leakage is called stress incontinence, and in pregnancy is due to the weight of your baby pushing down on your pelvic floor. You can help prevent stress

LEG CRAMPS

Leg cramps are extremely common during pregnancy and generally occur during the night. You can be woken up by a cramping pain, generally in one of your calf muscles or in the feet. The pain can be quite severe or come in spasms as the muscles cramp. It is not clear why cramps are more common in pregnancy, although theories include dehydration or salt imbalances. If you do get a cramp, try and stretch out the muscle to relieve the discomfort. Although painful, cramps are not dangerous. However, see your doctor if you have continuous or severe leg pain, with or without swelling, to check you have not developed a blood clot (deep vein thrombosis).

incontinence from worsening and improve your symptoms by doing pelvic floor exercises daily (for more information see Week 14).

Gestational diabetes

Gestational diabetes is diabetes that occurs during pregnancy in women who did not have diabetes before becoming pregnant. It is relatively common, affecting 1–3 per cent of pregnancies, and generally resolves after the baby has been born. You are at a higher risk of developing gestational diabetes if you have a previous history of it, are overweight, have a family history of diabetes, or if you have previously had a very large baby or a stillbirth.

Pregnancy hormones mean that your body does not respond as well as usual to the hormone insulin, which controls the level of sugar in your blood. In gestational diabetes not enough insulin is being produced, or the body is not responding to it, so levels of sugar in the blood become high (hyperglycaemia). This has various effects such as producing a large baby, which may then have low blood sugar after it is born as the baby was responding to the high levels of sugar in the mother's blood by producing more insulin.

Gestational diabetes is generally treated with dietary changes, though insulin treatment may be required. If you have gestational diabetes you will be offered care by a hospital obstetrician, and you may be given extra ultrasound scans to see how the pregnancy is progressing. You may also be offered appointments with a dietitian. If you have required treatment with insulin during your pregnancy you will be placed on an insulin and fluid drip during your labour in order to control your blood sugar levels.

If you have developed gestational diabetes you are at increased risk of developing diabetes later in life, so you will be offered an oral glucose tolerance test (see page 168) six weeks after the birth. You should also have an annual fasting blood glucose check.

SEX IN THE THIRD TRIMESTER

Many women enjoy an active and fulfilling sex life throughout their pregnancy. If there is a problem in your pregnancy, such as ruptured membranes or a very low-lying placenta, your antenatal team may advise you to avoid sex. However, there may be other ways in which you and your partner can enjoy some kind of sexual activity.

At this stage you may have to make some adjustments to avoid putting pressure on your bump. Positions where the woman is on top or squatting over her partner are possible even with a large bump, as are rear entry or side-by-side positions. Experimenting with different positions can be part of the fun!

You may notice that your baby moves when you are having intercourse. This does not mean your baby is distressed or aware of what is happening; he is probably just responding to the vibrations he can feel. After orgasm you may find that your uterus feels tight or that you have Braxton Hicks contractions (see Week 34). This is because the hormone released at orgasm is the same as the one that causes labour. However, sex will not bring on premature labour in a normal healthy pregnancy.

'WHEN SHOULD I FINISH WORK?'

If you are working while you are pregnant, there is no 'right' time to stop. You need to decide the time that is right for you. You can start your maternity leave from 11 weeks before your expected due date, so at Week 29 of your pregnancy that is any time from now on.

As your pregnancy progresses you may find work more tiring and would like a chance for some rest. You may wish to make preparations for the birth or spend time with your other children before the baby is born. This decision has to be weighed up against how much time you will then have with the baby after it has been born, as maternity leave does not last forever and a few months pass very quickly. Most women choose to have a few weeks at home before the baby is due, though of course no one can accurately predict when your baby will make its entrance!

'I stopped work at 36 weeks and was really glad to do so. It got really tiring in the last few weeks and I felt that I wanted to stop, relax and put all my focus on the baby, myself and my partner, my new family. It was strange to be stopping work, though, and knowing that I wouldn't be returning for at least six months – another step into the unknown. The lure of afternoon naps outweighs filing any day!' Rosie, 25

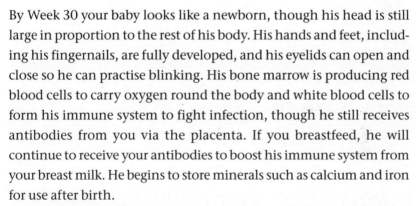

week 30

YOUR CHANGING BABY

By Week 30 your baby looks like a newborn, though his head is still large in proportion to the rest of his body. His hands and feet, including his fingernails, are fully developed, and his eyelids can open and close so he can practise blinking. His bone marrow is producing red blood cells to carry oxygen round the body and white blood cells to form his immune system to fight infection, though he still receives antibodies from you via the placenta. If you breastfeed, he will continue to receive your antibodies to boost his immune system from your breast milk. He begins to store minerals such as calcium and iron for use after birth.

He has now laid down enough fat under his skin to begin to control his own body temperature. This fat also makes his skin appear less wrinkled. He will use this fat after birth to keep him warm and supply him with energy while he waits for your milk supply and feeding to be established.

His brain and nervous system continue to develop and he spends a lot of his time asleep. When he is awake he moves around, stretching and kicking against the sides of your uterus, though there is less room for acrobatics as he gets bigger in proportion to the space in your womb.

At this point there is roughly 1.5 litres (2½ pints) of amniotic fluid around your baby. Your placenta is still growing and now weighs about 450 grams (1 pound). The average foetus measures approximately 40 centimetres (1 foot 3 inches) in length and weighs about 1.3–1.4 kilograms (3 pounds). For the next eight weeks or so he will put on around half a pound (200 grams) a week.

'I feel kicks all over the place – at the top, at the bottom, in the middle, everywhere. I think he must be doing somersaults and the splits in there! I feel them a lot at night, and if I stay still I can actually see my bump move as he moves inside. Occasionally I get a sharp kick under the ribs that makes me catch my breath but generally I love it; it's a reminder that he's in there – as if I could forget!' Hannah, 31

YOUR CHANGING BODY

Your uterus continues to increase in size and now reaches 10 centimetres (4 inches) above your belly button, about 30 centimetres (1 foot) in height. The hormone progesterone has helped your blood vessels to dilate and relax as much as possible, to cope with the increased blood volume and output from your heart without raising your blood pressure. From Week 30 onwards your blood vessels cannot dilate any further, though your blood volume will continue to rise. This means that your blood pressure, which has been lower than normal throughout your pregnancy, will gradually begin to rise back to pre-pregnancy levels. However, this increase should be gradual, and your blood pressure should still not be raised.

VAGINAL DISCHARGE

Women all have differing amounts of vaginal discharge. Even in the same woman the amount of discharge will vary during her menstrual cycle. Vaginal discharge increases in pregnancy from about the second trimester. This should look and smell like your normal vaginal secretions – clear or white in colour. If your discharge changes, for example becoming thick, smelly, very watery and profuse or changing colour, you should see your doctor who will examine you and take swabs to see if you have developed an infection. The examination is not risky for the baby. It is important to be checked out as some vaginal infections, such as bacterial vaginosis (also called BV), may increase the risk of premature labour unless treated with antibiotics.

Thrush

If your discharge has become thick, white and lumpy, sometimes described as 'cottage cheese', you may have developed thrush, especially if you are also itchy. Thrush is an overgrowth of a yeast called *Candida* that we all carry in our genital area, even when we are healthy. Candidal infections are common in pregnancy as hormones make your vagina less acidic, allowing the yeast to grow much more than normal.

Thrush does not increase your risk of going into premature labour, though it should be treated before you go into labour as otherwise there is a small risk of the baby catching it as it is born. It is easily treatable (both for you and if a baby does catch it), with either a tablet or a pessary inserted into the vagina. These medicines contain an antifungal to kill the yeast. They can be bought over the counter and are safe for use in pregnancy (though always tell your pharmacist that you are pregnant). You can also obtain a cream containing the same antifungal which can be used to relieve some of the itching associated with thrush. If using the pessary does not work, your doctor can try other medication. You will be examined to check that it is thrush, and swabs will be taken to see if the yeast is resistant to any medicines.

To prevent getting thrush wear cotton underwear to allow your skin to breathe. Make sure that you always wipe yourself from front to back after going to the toilet, whether it is to urinate or open your bowels, to avoid transferring bacteria from your anus to your vagina (this will also help prevent urinary tract infections). Do not use bubble bath, strong soap or feminine hygiene products as they may disrupt the normal balance of healthy bacteria and allow the yeast to overgrow.

'WHY AM I LEAKING FLUID FROM DOWN BELOW?'

It can be difficult to distinguish urine from amniotic fluid as they are both clear liquids. Some women may leak urine towards the end of their pregnancy. This can generally be prevented by doing regular pelvic floor exercises (see page 91). A leak of amniotic fluid is not normal and you would need to be examined and closely monitored by your doctor. If you only leak when you cough, laugh or jump up and down you may be leaking urine, but you should still be checked out. Your doctor will examine you to see if they can see a pool of liquid in the vagina, which would indicate that the liquid is amniotic fluid. If that is the case then your waters may have broken. Depending on the stage of your pregnancy, different action may be taken ranging from 'wait and see' to antibiotics or induction of labour.

EXERCISE IN THE THIRD TRIMESTER

You can continue to exercise during your final trimester, right up until you give birth. You will probably have to change the kind of exercise you do; after all, it is difficult to do gymnastics with a big bump affecting your centre of gravity. In general, women give up very strenuous exercise but you can still get your heart rate up and feel that you are working out. Be aware of your own limits, though, and don't push them.

EVERYONE'S GOT AN OPINION!

The later stages of pregnancy are difficult to conceal – your bump gives it away! Something that is hugely personal and special to you is common knowledge to everyone around you. Pregnancy is a curious state in that you may find that strangers or people you barely know ask to touch or stroke your bump. This can feel intrusive, as can the constant questioning about your pregnancy. People are very willing to give you advice, wanted or otherwise, about their own pregnancy and child-rearing experiences. Some women may revel in the attention, though it may make others feel uncomfortable. If you are feeling embarrassed or uncomfortable then tactfully say so, or try to change the subject. At the same time try to remember that people are not trying to make you feel uncomfortable; rather they think they are helping!

Lifting weights is not advisable but you can continue doing aerobic exercise, though you may find a brisk walk easier than a sprint! You can carry on with exercise such as yoga or Pilates, though again you may have to adjust the poses to compensate for your bump. Swimming is excellent exercise, especially in the third trimester (for more information see Week 33).

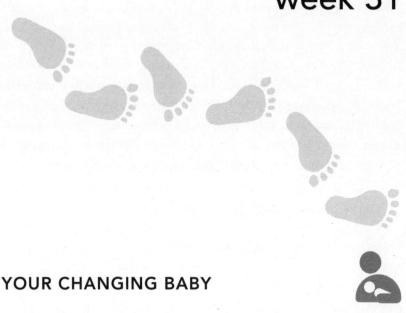

week 31

YOUR CHANGING BABY

Your baby's limbs are continuing to lengthen and he now has the proportions of a newborn baby. He will carry on growing and putting on weight, and his organs will continue to mature. His digestive system is functioning: his liver is producing bile to help him digest fats, and his pancreas is producing hormones to help control his blood sugar levels. His kidneys work to filter his blood and produce urine, which is stored in the bladder before being urinated into the amniotic fluid.

The adrenal glands on top of his kidneys now produce the hormone cortisol. This has many roles in the body, including helping in the production of surfactant and therefore the maturation of his lungs. If you were to go into labour early you might be given a steroid injection to help your baby's lungs.

He continues to gain muscle mass and to practise moving, kicking and stretching. You may even be able to see your bump moving as he moves around inside. Women often report that their babies move around a lot when they are relaxing in the bath. Let your partner and other children feel the kicking to keep them involved. The average foetus measures 41–42 centimetres (1 foot 4 inches) in length and weighs 1.5–1.6 kilograms (3 pounds 7 ounces).

YOUR CHANGING BODY

You might feel that you are sweating more than normal. This is because the increased blood flow to your skin makes you feel hot, and sweating is the body's natural response to feeling hot as it cools the body. The increased blood supply to the skin may also make the palms of your hands and soles of your feet look red, a condition called palmar erythema. This is normal, though it does not occur in all women, and the skin generally returns to normal after delivery.

Carpal tunnel syndrome

Carpal tunnel syndrome is more common in pregnant women. You may notice that you get pins and needles or a tingling or numb sensation in your fingers, generally your thumb and first two fingers. These fingers can also feel weak. The nerves, tendons and ligaments to your hands run through a structure called the carpal tunnel in your wrist. In pregnancy, fluid retention may make this structure swell and put pressure on the nerve as it enters your hand, causing the symptoms of tingling. As the fluid is reabsorbed and lost in the six weeks or so after delivery the symptoms should resolve. If it is causing you

ANTENATAL APPOINTMENT

If this is your first pregnancy you will be offered an antenatal appointment at around 31 weeks. You will be examined as usual and have the opportunity to discuss any concerns. The results of the blood tests taken at 28 weeks should be discussed with you.

discomfort your doctor may be able to refer you to a physiotherapist for a splint to help with the symptoms.

BUYING FOR BABY

Walking into a baby or nursery shop can be both confusing and intimidating as you are bombarded with information, and it can feel like you absolutely, desperately have to have one of everything, even though the costs are mounting rapidly. Remember that your baby won't know whether it is sleeping in the most fashionable (and often most expensive) pram or not! If you are looking for cheaper ways to kit out your nursery contact your local National Childbirth Trust (NCT) group who may be able to inform you if there is a second-hand sale in your area, or ask friends or family for items you can borrow. If you are using second-hand equipment you should always purchase a new mattress for your cot. You should not use a second-hand car seat as even the smallest of car accidents can cause damage to the seat.

As well as the items listed below, some parents purchase other equipment such as baby monitors, baby slings and a mobile. Remember, after the baby is born you may receive lots of gifts, and if not you will still be able to get out of the house to buy the extra things you need.

Sleeping

Many parents opt for a Moses basket, which will last for a few months before transferring the baby into a cot or cot bed. The advantage of a Moses basket is that it is relatively inexpensive and easily portable. You can set one up in your bedroom without taking up a lot of space. The disadvantage is that your baby will outgrow it in a few months. An alternative is a crib, a small rocking cot. These are generally more expensive and, again, only last a few months.

When buying a cot or cot bed make sure that you can work the cot sides and know how to adjust the base so that it can be lowered when your baby can stand up! Whatever you choose, you will need some bedding: sheets and blankets. Babies should not use duvets or pillows. Some parents prefer to purchase sleeping bags made of cotton or flannel that keep the baby warm without the risk of them pulling the covers over their heads.

'I went shopping for the baby's cot bedding and thought it would be relatively simple, but I got there and was bombarded by an entire wall of sheets – different colours, different materials, and sizes ranging from Moses baskets to beds. I just wanted some sheets – not ones with alarms or cartoon animals I didn't even recognise! Thankfully, a very nice shop assistant helped me out and now we are perfectly stocked, waiting for baby to arrive.' Suzanne, 36

Bathing

At first, you will probably be able to bath your baby in your bathroom sink. When they outgrow this you can bath them in your bath. Many parents prefer to purchase a baby bath, a small bathtub in which it may be easier to hold your baby. There are also various bath seats on the market which may make it easier to bath your baby as their weight (and initially their head) is supported. Whatever you choose, you will need to have some towels for your baby, though these don't have to be special 'baby towels' – a small towel of your own would be fine.

Changing

You will need to buy nappies, whether you aim to use disposable or washable ones. If you are using disposables don't stock up with months' worth of nappies in the smallest size as you may find that, at least initially, your baby grows rapidly and needs to have different nappy sizes.

If you intend to wash your nappies you will need terry towelling squares, muslin or disposable liners and safety pins, and you may wish to buy waterproof outer pants. Some disposables are handy when travelling or on holiday or for emergencies when everything is in the washing machine! You will need to purchase enough so that you can change your baby's nappies around eight to ten times per day without having to do washing daily. You could wash the nappies yourself or use a nappy laundering service.

You will also need some nappy cream, cotton wool for washing and some nappy sacks. You can use baby wipes, though cotton wool and water are just as good and may even be kinder to baby's skin. A nappy wrapper or unit is a container which wraps and stores used nappies in a plastic fragranced wrapper (which then looks like a sausage of nappies), sealing in smells so that you don't have to empty the dustbin so regularly, though this is not essential. Many women purchase a changing bag in which to store spare nappies, bottles and so on when they are out and about, though you can use any bag you already have at home.

You may also wish to purchase a changing table or chest of drawers with a changing area on the top. Some people feel that these are not necessary and changing your baby on the floor is safest. Changing mats can be purchased cheaply and mean that you won't be scrubbing urine off your carpet if there is an accident!

Car seats

If you travel by car you will need to purchase a car seat. In the UK there are strict legal guidelines regarding car seats for children, and you will need to purchase different seats as your child grows. Go to a store and ask the assistant to fit a seat into your car so that you can guarantee the seat is appropriate and safe for your car. Initially all babies travel rear facing; as they get older they will need a forward

THINGS TO BUY

Below is a suggested shopping list. The items with an asterisk beside them could be considered essential.

Sleeping:
* Moses basket/crib and/or cot/cot bed
* Mattress
* 4 bottom-fitted or flat sheets
* 4 blankets
2 baby sleeping bags
Baby monitor
Cot mobile

Changing:
* Nappies – disposable or washable
* Nappy cream
* Changing mat
Changing table/dresser
Nappy bin/wrapper/disposal unit
Nappy sacks

Bath time:
* Towels
* Wash cloths/sponge
* Baby-safe nail scissors
Hairbrush/comb
Baby bath
Bath seat/support

Baby clothes:
* 6–8 vests
* 6–8 all-in-one babygros (generally incorporating
  both socks and scratch-mitts)
* Hat
* Cardigan
Outdoor suit – depending on the season

Bottle feeding:
*Sterilising unit or tablets
*4–6 bottles and teats
*Bottle cleaning brush
* Muslin cloths (to protect your clothes when burping
  baby)
Bottle warmer (though a Pyrex jug of hot water is
fine)

Breastfeeding:
* Muslin cloths (to protect your clothes when burping
  baby)
Breast pump

Travel:
* Buggy/pram
Sling

Playtime:
Bouncing cradle
Mobile
Toys
Baby activity playmat/gym

facing seat. Some seats will transfer from being rear facing to forward facing. If you are leaving the hospital in a car you will need someone to bring the seat to hospital on the day you are leaving.

Buggies

You will probably wish to purchase a pushchair, buggy or pram, and there is a wide variety of options available. A pushchair that can lie flat is a good idea if your baby will be in it for long periods as lying flat is the best position for his spine and breathing.

Before you buy think about your lifestyle and what you intend to do with your buggy: do you live in a rural area and need something that can cope with not being on a smooth pavement? Do you live in a top-floor flat without a lift so will have to carry the buggy a lot? Do you travel by public transport and need something light and portable? Can you fit it in the boot of your car? Ask a shop assistant to demonstrate how the buggy works, and practise putting it up and down in the shop so that you will know how it functions before you take it home.

Of all the accessories that are available, probably the most essential is a rain cover for the buggy. Other accessories include parasols or sunshades and special blankets or warm coverings (often called cosytoes).

Clothing

You may receive lots of clothing gifts once your baby is born but make sure you have got the basics: vests, babygros, a cardigan or jacket and a hat. Babies are not very good at controlling their body temperature so generally need an extra layer to keep them warm, though it is important that they are not so well wrapped up that they get over-heated. Choose vests and clothes with wide or envelope-style necks so it is easy to put them on over your baby's head. You may wish to choose simple clothes that are easy to wash and throw in the tumble dryer as you will be busy after the birth!

Feeding

Breast is most certainly best, and with support the majority of women will find that they can breastfeed. Understandably, many women worry about whether or not they will be able to feed but a midwife or breastfeeding counsellor will show you. If you are intending to breastfeed a breast pump may be useful so you can express milk. Some women who are intending to breastfeed choose to purchase some bottles and formula milk, just in case.

If you don't think you will breastfeed (though it's always worth giving it a good go) you will need to purchase a sterilising unit which can work using steam or a sterilising agent. Many come with some bottles, though you will probably need to buy extra bottles and teats. You will also need a supply of formula milk. Formula milks are based on cow's milk and then modified to be as close to breast milk as possible. Which brand you choose is up to both you and your baby as they taste slightly different and your baby may develop a preference.

DIET IN THE THIRD TRIMESTER

During the third trimester your body will need approximately 200–300 extra calories per day. Two pieces of toast with butter is approximately 250–300 calories, so the extra amount is not actually very much, just a snack. You will probably find that you need to eat small amounts regularly as your stomach is smaller than normal due to your expanding uterus.

Continue to try and eat a healthy and varied diet. Make sure that you are drinking enough fluids, even though you need to go to the toilet a lot! On average, women gain 0.5–1 kilogram (1–2 pounds) per week during the third trimester, though this weight gain tends to slow down and may be minimal in the last few weeks of pregnancy.

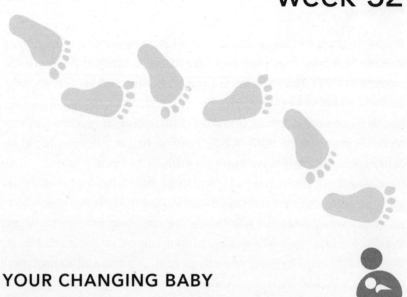

week 32

YOUR CHANGING BABY

You may feel that your baby is moving differently than previously. For example, you may feel shuffles or nudges as opposed to huge kicks or somersaults. This is because it is beginning to get a bit cramped in the womb. Although these movements may differ in quality, the pattern or number will stay the same.

His lungs continue to mature and he exercises them by practising breathing. The testicles in boys descend from the groin into the scrotum; this keeps them slightly cooler than the rest of the body and aids sperm production. Some babies settle into a cephalic or head-down presentation at this stage, ready for birth. Approximately 25 per cent of babies will be breech – bottom or feet down – at this stage; however, only about 3–4 per cent of babies are breech by 37 weeks, or term, because there is still enough room for him to turn around.

He now has enough control to move his head from side to side. He continues to grow hair, though how much hair he will have on his head at birth varies from baby to baby. The average foetus measures 42–43 centimetres (1 foot 5 inches) in length and weighs about 1.7 kilograms (3 pounds 12 ounces).

YOUR CHANGING BODY

The average woman notices that her breasts change and grow significantly during the first trimester. This growth then tends to slow off until the third trimester, when breasts continue to increase in size due to the effects of pregnancy hormones. Your breasts may feel heavier, can be tender and may also look different (apart from the obvious increase in size), with darker nipples and areolae (the coloured area around the nipple). You may have also noticed that you have prominent visible blue veins on your breasts, reflecting the increased blood supply to your breasts during pregnancy. You should get your breasts measured at least every four weeks during pregnancy, more if you feel that your bras are not fitting, so that you are wearing the correct bra to give your breasts adequate support. (For more information about bras in pregnancy see Week 6.)

Various hormones in pregnancy, such as human placental lactogen and prolactin, act on the breasts to prepare them for breastfeeding. However, no milk is produced yet as the high levels of oestrogen and progesterone from the placenta block milk secretion. After labour, when the placenta has been delivered, the change in hormone levels allows the prolactin to take effect so milk secretion starts.

Some women notice that their breasts leak a clear fluid during the last trimester of pregnancy. This is called colostrum, the substance your baby will drink for the first few days of its life, while it is waiting for your milk to come in. Other women do not notice any leakage, or only notice it at certain points, such as during or after sex. Leaking or not leaking colostrum during pregnancy is not a cause for concern.

PREMATURE LABOUR

A premature delivery is one that occurs before 37 weeks' gestation. If you are carrying a multiple pregnancy, such as twins or triplets, it is more likely that they will deliver early. Approximately 50 per cent of

'I CAN'T SLEEP!'

Many women find that their sleep is disturbed, especially during the later stages of pregnancy. This is often because it is difficult to get comfortable, and you may be waking up in the night to go to the bathroom. It can also be difficult to 'switch off' and relax as your mind may be full of lists or concerns, or even just thoughts about your baby and the weeks ahead.

Your bump makes it impossible to sleep on your front. Although you may be comfortable lying on your back, this position should be avoided as the weight of your bump can press on the large vessels which return blood to the heart. This can make you feel dizzy and even reduce the blood flow (and therefore oxygen supply) to your baby. So, if you do like to lie on your back then make sure you are propped up with lots of pillows behind your back and head, almost into a semi-sitting position. Lying on your side is a safe position; you may find it more comfortable if you use a pillow to support your bump and/or between your knees. Moving around in the bed at night can become quite cumbersome as you get bigger.

Many women also report that they dream vividly during pregnancy, and that these dreams can often be disturbing or frightening in nature. Perhaps women feel they are dreaming more because they wake up more often in the night; this means they are more likely to wake up during the dreaming phase of the sleep cycle and remember their dreams. Dreams are one way your subconscious deals with your emotions. Finally, nights of disturbed sleep may make you even more tired during the day so rest when you can and, if possible, take power naps during the daytime.

twin pregnancies will deliver prematurely. Multiple pregnancies also tend to produce smaller babies.

The earlier the gestation at which the baby is born the more likely it is to need medical help; therefore doctors try to keep babies inside the womb for as long as possible. If your waters break or contractions start before 37 weeks it is important that you go into hospital straight away to be examined. If your waters break it means that the membranes around the baby have ruptured. Even if labour does not start there is a risk of infection to the baby so you will be put on antibiotics. If you start showing signs of infection, such as a fever, your doctors will induce you or deliver the baby by Caesarean as the risk of infection may become greater than the risk of early delivery.

If you start having premature contractions you may be offered a special swab of the cervix to test for a substance called fibronectin. This can assess the likelihood of preterm labour. If the swabs are negative, preterm labour is unlikely so no treatment is given. If the swabs are positive, preterm labour is likely so treatment in the form of steroids and medication to relax the uterus is given.

Your antenatal team may give you a drip containing a medicine to relax the uterus. They may also give you injections of steroids to help your baby's lungs to mature; this tends to be given between 24 and 34 weeks' gestation as after this point the lungs are usually well developed. The medication to relax the uterus may stop labour. If labour is well established it may not be effective, though the steroids should hopefully have time to take effect in your baby. The injection of steroids is effective after 24 hours so the medication to relax the uterus (also called tocolysis) is generally stopped 24–48 hours after giving the first steroid injection.

Unless there are concerns that the baby needs to be delivered rapidly you should be able to deliver vaginally. You may need a Caesarean delivery if, for example, you are carrying twins and one is in a transverse position. Midwives, obstetric doctors and neonatal paediatricians may be present at the birth, and there is often a lot of medical equipment in the room, which can seem daunting. However, ensuring that equipment for every eventuality is easily available gives you and your baby the best care.

'Luke was born early, at 32 weeks. We were out for dinner with friends when my waters broke. We went to hospital straight away. There were no problems with the labour itself, which was really quick, but I remember that there were a lot of people in the room – midwives, obstetric doctors and paediatric doctors and nurses. As soon as he was born they whipped him off to check him over; at first he needed a little help with his breathing and went to the special baby unit. He stayed there for a few weeks; as he was so small he needed help feeding. Of course it was hard but I went there every day and sat with him, held him, loved him, and those few weeks passed and we went home. Nine months later he is a happy, healthy, bouncing boy and you would never know anything had happened.' Kate, 33

Depending on how early the baby is, he may need medical intervention in the special care baby unit or neonatal intensive care. If so, your baby will be looked after by a team of nurses and neonatal paediatricians. Intervention can range from help with breathing to help with feeding if your baby does not have a well-developed suckling reflex or digestive system.

Delivering a baby or babies prematurely is a very stressful time. You may have various anxieties, not just about the health of your newborn but also about not having everything ready at home. If your baby is in the neonatal unit you may also be very anxious that you will not be able to be close to him straight away. However, as parents, you will be able to spend lots of time in the unit and will have the opportunity to breastfeed and give plenty of cuddles, so you will be able to bond with your baby.

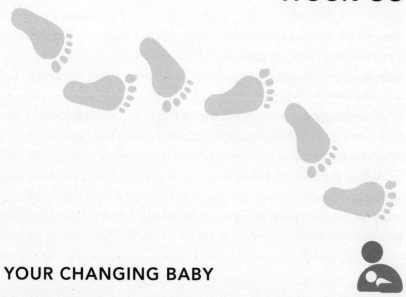

week 33

YOUR CHANGING BABY

Your baby's bones continue to harden, but the bones of his skull remain malleable and not fully joined up; this allows them to move and pass over one another so that he can travel through the birth canal. His fingernails continue to grow; by now they reach the ends of his fingertips or even further, and though his nails are still soft he may be able to scratch himself before he is born.

The lanugo hair, which covered his body to protect him from the effects of continual immersion, begins to be lost. By now he is drinking about a pint of amniotic fluid a day and urinating it back out again. He continues to lay down fat and also stores glycogen in his liver; both these can be used as an energy source after birth. His skin begins to look less red and wrinkly. The average foetus measures approximately 44 centimetres (1 foot 5 inches) in length and weighs about 1.9–2 kilograms (4 pounds 5 ounces). About half of your weekly weight gain from now on will be from your baby growing.

YOUR CHANGING BODY

You might have noticed that your fingers, hands, ankles and legs have become swollen. Slight swelling is common in pregnancy; the volume of fluid in your body has increased to such an extent that you will probably be retaining water. To try and relieve any swelling in your ankles avoid standing still for long periods; moving around will help your leg muscles to pump some of the fluid back to your heart. Sitting with your legs up can also help to relieve the swelling. Not all women have swelling but if you notice that your face is puffy and swollen, or if the amount of swelling you have in your extremities increases rapidly, go to your doctor as this may signify pre-eclampsia (for more information see page 155).

Varicose veins and vulval varicosities

Varicose veins are enlarged veins seen just under the surface of the skin. They are often twisted or bulging, bluish or purple, and are extremely common in pregnancy. All your blood vessels will have dilated during pregnancy to cope with your increased blood volume without causing a rise in blood pressure. The weight of your bump also puts pressure on the veins in your pelvis, making it difficult for the blood to flow back to your heart. The bump acts like a road block – just as the cars back up on the road leading up to a road block, there is an increased backflow of blood in the veins in your legs. The valves in your veins cannot cope with this extra pressure so the smaller, dependent veins fill up and cause varicose veins. These can be small, such as thread veins, or large.

Generally, varicose veins do not cause any problem apart from the fact that some women may consider them unsightly, but they can cause aching or throbbing legs. Keep mobile, as the action of your calf muscles working helps pump blood through the vessels. Compression stockings (available from pharmacies) may improve symptoms as they help the blood flow back to the heart. Varicose veins generally resolve after delivery but they can remain.

Varicose veins can also occur in your vulva, for the same reasons as described above. In some women these may cause discomfort, such as when sitting down. Vulval varicosities usually resolve after delivery, though very rarely they can bleed during labour. If you do develop vulval varicosities, simple things like sitting on a (wrapped) ice pack may help with the discomfort. Haemorrhoids are dilated veins in the anus (for more information see Week 28).

YOUR BIRTH PLAN

You may have started to consider a birth plan, or have talked about it with your midwife or antenatal team. A birth plan is a way of thinking about what you would like to happen in your labour, a method of discussing various options and situations that may arise. It is important to remember that things do not always fit the plan. Your circumstances may change and it can be difficult to predict what you would want, or how you may feel, in any given situation.

Birth plans are a way of communicating your wishes to your midwives and doctors but it is important to try and keep an open mind. If you are very rigid about what 'must' or 'must not' happen, you may find it difficult to cope if the situation changes. For example, in an ideal world you may wish to avoid a Caesarean, but if an emergency arises and the doctors need to deliver the baby quickly to ensure its safety, a Caesarean may be the best option. Your team will of course try to comply with your wishes while ensuring your well-being and your baby's safe delivery.

Topics you may wish to discuss or include in your birth plan are listed below. (For more information about each of these topics see 'Labour', pages 245–292.)

- Who would you like to be present at the birth – for example your partner, your mother or a friend?
- Do you want your midwife to offer you pain relief?

- What kinds of pain relief would you consider? Gas and air, pethidine, epidural?
- Would you like to keep mobile during labour? Use a birthing ball?
- Would you like to use a birthing pool? For pain relief in the early stages of labour or for the actual delivery?
- Do you mind if a medical or midwifery student is present during your delivery, or even delivers your baby (under supervision)?
- If your midwife/doctor feels it necessary, would you be prepared to have your membranes ruptured or given medication to speed up your contractions?
- If recommended, would you consider an episiotomy?
- Do you want the baby to be placed 'skin to skin' on your tummy or into your arms straight after delivery? Would you like the midwife to check the baby before giving it to you?
- Would you or your partner like to cut the umbilical cord?
- Would you agree to an injection of a medication to speed up the delivery of the placenta?

You may have other ideas about what you would like for your labour. For example, you may want to have music playing. Think about your options and discuss them with your team. You could involve your partner in these discussions as he may have opinions about certain topics, but also so that he is aware of your wishes and can speak out for you during labour if you feel unable to do so.

No birth plan is set in stone. Just as your medical or midwifery team may advise you to change the plan if circumstances dictate it, you can also change your mind. Just speak to your midwife at the time.

PERINEAL MASSAGE

Perineal massage may help to increase the elasticity of the skin in your perineum – the area between your vagina and anus. It may help prevent tearing or decrease the need for an episiotomy (see page 277) during delivery. Massaging this area promotes blood flow to the perineum, which can speed up healing after labour. It also helps you become aware of the stretching sensation in this region which you will feel as the skin becomes stretched by the baby's head during delivery.

'CAN I GO SWIMMING?'

By this point in your pregnancy you will probably be finding it difficult to exercise. Do remember, though, that even the most mundane activities can be forms of exercise: climbing stairs, walking to the bus stop, carrying the shopping and doing the housework all count. Swimming is fantastic during pregnancy as the water supports your weight without putting any stress on your joints. It is a great cardiovascular exercise, getting your blood pumping around your body, and so can help with water retention or swollen ankles. Cardiovascular exercise also builds your fitness endurance levels, which will help you prepare for the work of labour.

Swimming uses all the major muscle groups so helps increase your muscle tone. Again, this will help you prepare for labour. Good muscle tone has the added benefit of helping you return to your pre-pregnancy weight. Although you can choose any swimming stroke during pregnancy, even just floating with the water buoying you up can be very relaxing. Saunas, Jacuzzis and steam rooms should be avoided in pregnancy.

Starting perineal massage about four to six weeks before your expected delivery date should be sufficient and can be performed daily. Do not do perineal massage if you have an infection such as thrush or herpes to prevent the infection spreading. Firstly, wash your hands and use a water-based lubricant such as KY jelly, or an unscented oil such as olive oil or sweet almond oil, on your hands. Sit comfortably with your legs apart. The first few times you may wish to use a mirror so you can see what you are doing. Using one or two thumbs place them about 2–3 centimetres (about half your thumb's length) inside your vagina and press downwards and sideways until you feel a stretching sensation. You can hold this stretch for a minute or two and then gently massage the lower section of the vagina in a 'U' shape, applying pressure downwards and sideways. To decrease the risk of a urine infection only massage the lower half of the vagina (nearest your anus) to avoid touching your urethra (tube which connects to your bladder). Your partner could help and perform the perineal massage using the same technique, but using his index finger/s instead of his thumb/s.

> 'I was never a big fan of swimming before I was pregnant, what with all the changing, wet hair and communal changing rooms, but now I love it. When I'm out I feel heavy with a huge belly but in there I am light as the water supports me. The same is true in a warm bath, but there I look a bit like a hippo as my breasts and bump stick out of the water!' Gaby, 27

FOR FATHERS

As your partner gets larger during the later stages of the pregnancy you may find yourself having to help her more than previously. This assistance can mean anything from helping heave her up off the sofa to tying her shoes if she can't reach over her bump. Often support is not just practical but emotional. It can be a two-way process as both of you may have anxieties about the upcoming labour and then parenthood.

From a practical point of view the third trimester is often a time when fathers-to-be are asked to become handymen, decorating nurseries or building cots. Although your wife may well be capable of these things, the third trimester of pregnancy isn't really the time for her to be hanging off a ladder painting the ceiling! Preparing a space for your child, even if that is simply moving objects so there is room for a Moses basket in your room, does help make things real, and can help prepare you emotionally for bringing a baby home. You might like to learn to fit the car seat, and to set up and collapse your buggy or pram – these things may sound easy but often have extremely complicated instructions so get prepared so you aren't struggling with a newborn! Make sure that your boss at your workplace knows that your partner is pregnant and about any plans you have for paternity leave (for more information see page 130).

'How does one little baby need so much stuff? Bags and bags of towels and sheets and nappies and yet more nappies! One afternoon I helped unpack this mountain of bags and found myself in awe of the vests – they were so small and soon there was going to be a baby in them. It really brought things home. The baby's coming now, and we're ready, or at least the clothes are!' Stuart, 34

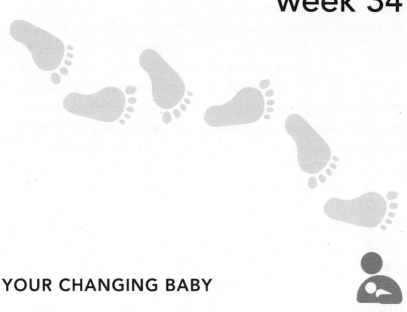

week 34

YOUR CHANGING BABY

Your baby's organs are now mature but the next few weeks are still important for further growth, weight gain and maturation. He carries on laying down fat in his abdomen and in his arms and legs; he may even have a little rounded tummy and his skin will look less wrinkly. This fat will help him control his body temperature and supply energy until feeding is well established.

His hearing is developed and he recognises your voice. You may feel that he is less active than previously as he has less room for movement; however, he will still be kicking and stretching regularly. The average foetus measures approximately 45 centimetres (1 foot 5½ inches) in length and weighs about 2.15–2.2 kilograms (4 pounds 12 ounces).

YOUR CHANGING BODY

Your brain produces a hormone called oxytocin from the pituitary gland. This is the hormone that makes your uterus contract during labour. During the final stages of your pregnancy the amount of receptors for oxytocin in your womb increase so that it can respond to the hormone during labour. As labour progresses, your dilating cervix further stimulates oxytocin production to increase your contractions. After the birth, the action of your baby suckling on your nipples during breastfeeding also stimulates the production of oxytocin, which then acts to contract your uterus back to its pre-pregnancy size; these contractions can be painful and are sometimes called 'after pains'.

During the late stages of pregnancy your bump has expanded so much that your belly button might pop out. Your belly button is a scar from the site at which you were connected to your umbilical cord when you were in the womb. If your navel has become inverted it can be quite prominent but should return to normal after delivery.

BRAXTON HICKS CONTRACTIONS

Braxton Hicks contractions are the practice contractions of your uterus as it prepares for labour. They also ensure that more blood goes into your placenta. You may have already been feeling some Braxton Hicks, and these become more common as your pregnancy enters its final stages.

These practice contractions are generally painless, starting at the top of your uterus and travelling downwards. They can feel like a tightening or hardening of your uterus that lasts for approximately 30 seconds and can be uncomfortable, especially towards the final weeks of your pregnancy. This is a good opportunity to try some of your relaxation techniques, such as a warm bath or back rub, as prac-tice for labour.

Braxton Hicks contractions are different from the true contrac-tions of labour in that they are painless and very irregular. Labour contractions increase in both strength and frequency as labour progresses. However, it may be difficult to distinguish Braxton Hicks contractions from the true contractions of labour, especially if this is your first pregnancy. If you do think you are in labour then phone or go into your labour ward to discuss your symptoms. You may be advised to go in to be examined.

> 'At first it was difficult to tell what was going on. I'd put my hand on my tummy and it would go completely hard; I felt a tightening sensation but it wasn't a pain. So I rang the labour ward who said they were probably Braxton Hicks but if they started getting regular or painful to come in. Just speaking to them reassured me, and sure enough they were right – they just stopped on their own.' Molly, 42

ANTENATAL APPOINTMENT

If you were not seen at 31 weeks the results of your last blood tests will be discussed at this appointment. Some units offer a further blood test to check that you have not become anaemic at this point. If your blood group is Rhesus negative you may be offered another injection of anti-D to prevent you building up antibodies, though some units now only give a single dose of anti-D (of a different dosage) at 28 weeks of pregnancy. You will be offered a further injection of anti-D if there is any bleeding in the pregnancy and after the delivery (for more information see Week 11).

If you had a 'low-lying placenta' at your 20-week scan you will be offered another ultrasound scan at 32–36 weeks. A low-lying placenta is where the placenta is in the lower section of the uterus, sometimes near or even covering the cervix. In the majority of cases a low-lying placenta will have risen up as the uterus grows during pregnancy. If your placenta is still low it is termed 'placenta praevia'. Depending on how close to the cervix the placenta is it may require special consideration during your care and labour; it can cause bleeding and

PLACENTA PRAEVIA

In placenta praevia the placenta is in the lower part of the womb and can cover the cervix. It is more likely to occur if you have had a previous placenta praevia or a previous Caesarean section, and in older mothers. It is graded according to how much of the placenta is covering the cervix:

- Grade I – the placenta is low but not covering the cervix
- Grade II – the placenta touches the opening of the cervix but does not cover it
- Grade III – the placenta partially covers the cervix
- Grade IV – the opening of the cervix is completely obstructed by the placenta

For women with grades I and II, the baby can be born vaginally. However, if grade III or IV is present the baby has to be born by Caesarean as the placenta is covering the cervix.

One of the risks of placenta praevia is bleeding, which is often painless and tends to occur at the end of the second trimester or in the last trimester of pregnancy. If you are diagnosed with placenta praevia you may be advised to avoid vigorous exercise and sex. If you are bleeding you should go to hospital for assessment.

you may require a Caesarean section. A low-lying placenta in the early stage of pregnancy is quite common, affecting about 20 per cent of women, but placenta praevia occurs in only 0.2 per cent of pregnancies, or 1 in 200 pregnancies, at full term.

During this appointment your doctor or midwife will begin to discuss labour and how to recognise that labour is starting (see Week 39). They may also discuss some of the options you would like to consider in your birth plan (see Week 33). Thinking about these issues early gives you time to make informed choices.

GROUP B STREPTOCOCCUS

Group B streptococcus (GBS) is a bacterium commonly carried in your intestines. Up to 30 per cent of women have this bacterium in their upper vagina. It generally causes no problems, though occasionally can provoke a urinary tract infection or a discharge from the vagina.

GBS can be a cause for concern during pregnancy because as the baby passes through the birth canal he may swallow or inhale some of the secretions and pick up the bacterium. This is uncommon, affecting 1 per cent of babies from at-risk mothers (see below), but can be extremely serious or even fatal, causing severe infections such as meningitis. The infection generally becomes apparent within the first 48 hours after birth. If the infection is found in the baby it can be treated with antibiotics.

Are pregnant women screened for GBS?

There is no national screening programme for GBS in the UK, which would involve taking a swab from the lower vagina. This is because you can have a positive swab one week and be negative the next, and vice versa. A positive swab simply means you are carrying the bacterium at that particular point in time, not that it will cause any problems. Treating a positive swab (as long as your waters haven't broken) does not reduce the risk of GBS in the baby. Therefore, pregnant women in the UK are not screened for GBS. However, women identified as having risk factors for GBS will be treated during labour (for more information see below), and any babies who become unwell soon after delivery will be tested and treated for the infection.

How are women identified for treatment?

Women with risk factors for GBS will have treatment during labour. Risk factors include:

- having a previous baby infected with GBS
- GBS identified on swabs during this pregnancy (these swabs may be taken for other reasons, such as suspected thrush)
- a urinary tract infection with GBS during the current pregnancy
- your waters breaking before you are term
- prolonged rupture of membranes – your waters break and you don't deliver within 18 hours
- premature labour (at less than 37 weeks)
- a fever of over 38°C during labour

Having GBS on a swab or with a urinary tract infection in a previous pregnancy does not mean that you will have treatment during this labour if you have no risk factors during this pregnancy.

'What happens if I have a risk factor for GBS?'

If you have a risk factor for GBS the treatment is with intravenous antibiotics during labour. Antibiotics are given every four hours, and two doses are needed for treatment to be considered complete. If your labour is between two and four hours long you will only have one dose of antibiotics; in this situation the treatment is considered suboptimal and so your baby will be closely monitored for 12 hours after delivery. If your labour is less than two hours long, the treatment will not be considered effective, even if you have had one dose of antibiotics. Your baby will therefore be monitored, have blood tests and receive intravenous antibiotics. If this is the case you and the baby will be in hospital for at least 48 hours. If you have a premature delivery your baby will have blood tests and intravenous antibiotics even if you have had adequate treatment during your labour as premature babies are more likely to become infected and unwell than those born at full term.

If you have a risk factor for GBS but are having an elective Caesarean section you will not need antibiotics as long as labour hasn't started before the Caesarean is performed. This is because the baby is protected in the womb from many infections, and during a Caesarean the baby does not pass through the vagina.

Why isn't GBS treated before labour starts?

Treating GBS with oral antibiotics during pregnancy is not considered effective. This is because 70 per cent of women treated with antibiotics during the third trimester of pregnancy will have GBS again within three weeks of treatment. So treating with oral antibiotics is no guarantee that you won't have GBS when you go into labour. The evidence in the UK is that giving antibiotics during labour decreases the number of newborns infected with GBS by about 75 per cent. Also, if everyone were treated with oral antibiotics, the bacterium would become resistant to antibiotics and the infection would become more difficult to treat.

THE NESTING INSTINCT

Many women describe a need or compulsion to get things done around the house during the final weeks of their pregnancy. It is extremely common to find heavily pregnant women absolutely insisting that they need to clean out their kitchen cupboards, repaint ceilings or sort out the loft, much to the surprise of their partner! Why these urges, or the nesting instinct, occur is not known, but it may be a way of preparing for labour and the upcoming changes in your life. In order to have the time and space to focus entirely on the job in hand – that is safely delivering and then looking after a newborn – perhaps women need to know that everything else is as organised as it can be.

'I turned into one of those crazy pregnant women. You know the ones – eight months pregnant and halfway up a ladder cleaning on top of the cupboards. But it was like I couldn't relax until everything was clean and perfect, ready for the baby to come. My husband said I was preparing for a siege!' Lisa, 29

'I CAN'T GET OFF THE SOFA WITHOUT HELP!'

To protect your back and to prevent straining your tummy muscles you will have to adapt how you bend down and get up to compensate for your bump. When bending down, bend at the knees to squat as opposed to bending at the waist. To get up from lying down safely, such as when getting out of bed, roll on to your side and then swing your legs over the edge of the bed. Then push yourself up to sitting using your arms. You should now be sitting on the edge of your bed and will be able to stand up easily. To get up from lying on the floor first lie on your side and bend your knees, then bring the knee that is beneath you, the knee that is closest to the floor, further up. Next, shift your weight on to your arms and the underside knee so that you can turn to be on all fours. You should then be able to stand up.

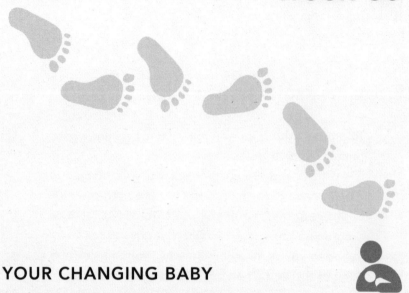

YOUR CHANGING BABY

Your baby is continuing to grow and prepare himself for birth. The amount of amniotic fluid in your womb may begin to decrease as your baby takes up most of the available space. He continues to gain weight rapidly: about 220 grams (half a pound) per week; about 30 grams (1 ounce) per day.

As he is getting larger there is less room for him to move around and you may notice that the movements feel different. They may be more like pushes than kicks, though the number of movements will still be the same. When he does move you may be able to see an indent of a foot through your bump! Your baby may have periods of activity and periods of sleep so you won't feel him moving all the time, though you should still feel movements regularly.

His lungs are almost fully developed and he now produces a hormone called cortisol to help them mature further. His intestine is full of meconium ready for his first bowel motion, which will be thick, sticky and greenish black. His nervous system continues to develop and his reflexes have become strong and co-ordinated: he can grasp, search for a nipple and suck; he is also now very responsive to sound, light and touch. You have about 1 litre (1¾ pints) of amniotic fluid and he is urinating about 500 millilitres (16 fluid ounces) per day. The average foetus measures approximately 46 centimetres (1 foot 6 inches) in length and weighs about 2.4 kilograms (5 pounds 4 ounces).

YOUR CHANGING BODY

By approximately the 35th week of pregnancy your blood volume will have reached its peak of about 7 or 8 litres (12½–14 pints). This dilution of your red blood cells in relation to your plasma volume can make you anaemic. This anaemia generally causes no problems as you still have more red blood cells than previously. However, your antenatal team will check your blood count, especially if you are feeling more tired or short of breath than you would expect. If you do have mild anaemia you may be advised to take iron tablets; if this is the case do not worry if your stool turns black as this is an effect of the tablets. Iron tablets may also make you constipated so be sure to eat lots of fruit and vegetables and drink plenty of water. If this doesn't help, your doctor will be able to prescribe a laxative which is safe in pregnancy. Iron tablets are best taken with some orange juice as the vitamin C in the juice helps your body to absorb the iron.

'My pelvis hurts, just under my bump'

Generalised backache is extremely common in pregnancy due to the extra strain put on your back muscles (for more information see page 144). However, if you experience severe lower back or pelvic pain you should see your doctor as it is also common to develop a specific condition during pregnancy such as those described below:

Pubic symphysis dysfunction
The pubic symphysis is the point on the front of your pelvis (the pubis) where the two halves of your pelvis join. Due to the effects of pregnancy hormones, the connective tissue in your pelvis relaxes and the two pubic bones can separate slightly and rub together when you

walk. This causes pain in your pelvis, just in front of your bladder. Ice packs may reduce any swelling and paracetamol can help with the pain. To help keep your pelvis together avoid moving your knees wide apart or straddling motions. Your doctor or midwife can also refer you to a physiotherapist for exercises and treatment. Some women require crutches to help them walk.

Sciatica

This is due to pressure on the sciatic nerve, which runs from the spinal cord in your back through your buttocks and down your legs. If the nerve is compressed it can lead to a constant or intermittent sharp, shooting pain in your lower back, buttocks or down your leg. Sometimes this can be associated with numbness or tingling in the leg, or even leg weakness.

Sacroiliac pain

Also called pelvic girdle dysfunction, this is pain generally felt in one or both of the buttocks. It occurs due to pregnancy hormones relaxing the ligaments of your pelvis, together with changes in your posture to compensate for the weight of your bump. As with pubic symphysis dysfunction (see above) this is relieved with paracetamol and may benefit from physiotherapy.

Coccygeal pain

The coccyx, often called the tailbone, is found at the bottom of the spine. Again, due to the effects of pregnancy hormones and the weight from your bump, this region can become painful. You will feel the pain at the very base of your spine or in the buttocks. Try to sit up straight and avoid slumping to take the pressure off your coccyx. Sitting on a soft pillow may help, as can exercises such as pelvic tilts (see Week 25).

Treatment

These conditions may need specific treatments, though simple measures such as ice packs or hot water bottles and paracetamol may be effective. Taking care to look after your back and doing back exercises regularly may help prevent such conditions. If they do develop and are severe, your doctor may refer you to a women's health physio-therapist for more directed therapy, such as giving you specific exercises to relieve the problem. For pubic symphysis dysfunction you may be given a brace (essentially a large piece of tubigrip) to wear over your bump and pelvis for support.

FEAR OF LABOUR

Most women are apprehensive about labour. Even if you have had a baby previously there is no way of predicting how the next delivery will be. Concerns range from being mildly anxious to panic attacks. Tokophobia is a phobia of childbirth. It can cause serious difficulties as women may want to have babies but may feel unable to do so as their fears relating to labour are so intense. If you feel that your anxieties are adversely affecting you, speak to your antenatal team, preferably as early in your pregnancy as possible. They may be able to reassure you, or if not, may refer you to a psychologist or therapist for treatment, such as cognitive behavioural therapy, to help with your fears.

Many women have concerns about how they will act during labour. They worry about various things such as screaming or shout-ing, being out of control or not looking their best. Rest assured that your midwives and doctors will not be fazed by a bit of groaning or shouting; after all, they are used to dealing with labouring women. Other women are concerned about passing a stool during pushing in labour; this can occur as there may be some stool in your rectum, but if it does your midwife will simply remove it and you probably won't even notice. Many women feel the need to open their bowels during the early stages of labour so in general the rectum is empty.

You may be concerned about going into labour in a public place – your waters breaking in a shop, for instance, or having the baby on a bus on the way to hospital. Such situations do arise, but are uncom-mon. The majority of women will be able to reach the hospital or birthing unit in time. Many women are concerned that their partner will not be able to get to them in time for the birth. Put your mind at rest by making plans for contacting your partner when you go into labour. Discuss what to do if he cannot get there quickly and what will happen to any other children while you are in labour.

Perhaps the most common concern is about your safety and the health and wellbeing of your baby. What will he look like? Will he be healthy? Will he be disfigured in some way? Try to remember that the aim of your antenatal and postnatal care is to keep you and your baby safe, and that everything necessary will be done in labour for you and your baby. Also remember that in the majority of cases mothers and babies are fine, happy and healthy, and that women have been giving birth all over the world for years without any intervention.

'I keep getting anxious whenever I think about going into labour – what if I can't contact my partner, what if I can't deal with the pain, what if something happens, what if the baby isn't okay? It is the feeling of not being in control and not knowing what is going to happen next that worries me. I spoke to my midwife and we went over everything that can happen during labour together. Knowing about my options really helped. It's happening, no matter what, so I am trying to relax about it!' Jade, 34

BREECH BABIES

A breech presentation is when your baby is buttocks or feet down, instead of head down, into the pelvis. The earlier on in your pregnancy that your baby is breech the more likely he is to turn head down as there will still be room in the uterus for turning. However, approximately 4 per cent of babies are breech at full term (after 37 weeks).

If you have a breech baby you may be offered external cephalic version (ECV) at approximately 37 weeks. ECV is a method whereby your doctor attempts to turn your baby by manipulating him through your abdomen. Generally you will be asked to come into the labour ward or maternity day unit for ECV and the baby's heart rate will be monitored both before and after the procedure, and if there are complications the baby may have to be delivered.

If your baby remains breech it is still possible to have a vaginal delivery, though complications are more common. A Caesarean section may be advised. Your doctor will advise you as to the safest method to deliver your baby, taking your wishes into account.

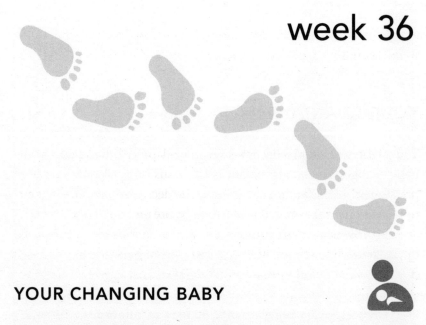

week 36

YOUR CHANGING BABY

Your baby continues to put on weight in preparation for life after birth. His body has become round and his arms and legs have filled out. The majority of babies are in the cephalic presentation – head down – though some may be in the breech position – bottom or feet down (see Week 35). The position your baby is in is unlikely to change before labour as there is simply not enough room for him to turn. You may feel your baby squirming or wriggling from side to side as he tries to get comfortable.

He may 'drop' or 'engage' as his head, or presenting part, moves further into the pelvis towards the birth canal. When this happens, his head is protected by the bones of your pelvis. If this is your first pregnancy, engagement can occur at any time from this point onwards; if you have had previous deliveries, engagement tends to occur later – it can happen just before you go into, or even during, labour. If you are carrying a multiple pregnancy, one of the babies may engage during the later stages of pregnancy; the second twin can only engage after the first is delivered, as there is only enough room for one head at a time in your pelvis!

The lungs continue to mature, though all his other organs are fully developed and functioning. The average foetus measures approximately 47–48 centimetres (1 foot 6½ inches) in length and weighs about 2.65—2.7 kilograms (5 pounds 14 ounces).

YOUR CHANGING BODY

You might notice that it becomes easier to take deep breaths once your baby engages or drops into your pelvis. This is because there is less pressure on your diaphragm and ribs. The decreased pressure in your upper abdomen also means that there is more room for your stomach and digestive system, so you may be able to eat more in one meal as opposed to having to eat little and often. However, as the baby's head descends it will compress your bladder, giving it even less room to expand and hold urine, so you will be going to the toilet more regularly, though only passing small amounts of urine at a time.

'I'm back to the toilet again. I spent most of the first trimester there, what with being sick and needing to wee all the time. This time there is no sickness but it feels like I go to the toilet every hour or so. It is quite annoying!' Farah, 24

'My bump has dropped!'

As your baby's head engages into your pelvis it can look and feel like your bump has dropped. The weight of your baby and uterus is now held in a lower position than previously so you have to compensate further for the change in your centre of gravity. This is done by subconsciously leaning back, even further than you already have been doing. The changes in your posture, combined with the laxity of your ligaments due to the effects of your pregnancy hormones, mean that there is even more strain placed on your lower back, often causing backache. (For more information about backache in pregnancy, and exercises to prevent and relieve it, see Weeks 24, 27 and 35.)

ANTENATAL APPOINTMENT

From 36 weeks onwards you will be offered antenatal appointments more regularly until the baby is born. They will take the same structure as previously, though it can be increasingly difficult to get your urine sample into the seemingly ever-shrinking pot as you can no longer see what you are doing over your bump!

Your doctor or midwife will feel your baby through your abdomen to assess its lie (whether it is vertical, horizontal or diagonal in position) and presentation (which part is nearest your pelvis, generally head or bottom). Now they will also palpate your bump to see whether or not your baby's head has engaged. The head is engaged when more than half of it (or three-fifths) is within the bony confines of your pelvis, so less than half (two-fifths) can still be felt through your bump. If your midwife can feel the shape of the whole head then it is not yet engaged. They will note how many fifths of the head they think can still be felt to decide whether or not the head is engaged. A further method of assessing head engagement is to do a manual vaginal examination, though this is not generally carried out.

Your antenatal team will also begin to discuss postnatal topics in order to plan for the future, including breastfeeding, newborn screening tests and newborn vitamin K. They will also inform you about the baby blues and postnatal depression so that you may be able to recognise it if you do need some help later on. (For more information on these topics see 'Labour' and 'The Postpartum Period'.)

YOUR HOSPITAL BAG

In general, you will have to bring everything you and your baby will need while in hospital, though if your delivery takes you by surprise the hospital should have some supplies!

What to pack

For you:
- Nightwear
- Underwear (including nursing bras)
- Dressing gown
- Slippers
- Towel
- Toiletries – toothbrush, toothpaste, deodorant, hairbrush, shampoo
- Maternity sanitary pads (special sanitary towels) – you will need these as you will bleed (like a period) after delivery, and you can buy them from pharmacies (for more information see 'The Post-partum Period')
- Breast pads and nipple cream (for more information see 'Breast-feeding', page 310)

For baby:
- Two to three vests
- Two to three babygros or sleepsuits
- Cardigan
- Hat
- Outdoor suit or something to go home in if it is cold
- Nappies
- Nappy sacks
- Cotton wool
- Nappy cream

You may choose to include other options such as comfortable daywear for yourself in case you need to stay in hospital and wish to get dressed, and a change of clothes for your partner. Snacks for yourself or your partner are often a good idea as you may get hungry during a long labour, or bring some change for a vending machine (though these rarely stock healthy choices!) Other items include a camera, video camera, music, earplugs, books and magazines. Items such as a TENS machine for pain relief (for more informtion see 'Labour') can be bought or hired. Don't forget a list of important contact numbers for all those people with whom you will want to share your news.

It can seem like a lot, as if you are packing for a two-week holiday! Remember that if you forget something you need, then your partner or a friend or family member should be able to go and get it for you. Finally, when it is time to go home from the hospital, you will need to bring your baby's car seat to the hospital if you are travelling by car.

YOGA

The cat-cow sequence described below can be useful to relieve lower backache, which is common in the later stages of pregnancy.

- Start on all fours with your tummy muscles drawn in, looking down at the floor. Your knees should be hip-width apart and your arms shoulder-width apart. Your elbows should be straight, and your hands should be on the floor with fingers facing forward. Keep your back flat, in the neutral pose.
- Inhale and tilt your tailbone down while tilting your head to the ceiling so your back arches.
- Exhale and move back to the centre, then downwards. Draw your tummy muscles into your spine and round your back the other way, tucking your bottom in and under. Your head should be bent and looking at the floor, with your chin tucked into your chest. This is the cat pose.
- Repeat by inhaling and arching your back, exhaling and rounding your back three or four times.

- Go into child's pose (see page 168) for one breath before repeating the sequence.
- If you feel there is too much pressure on your knees, put a folded blanket underneath them.

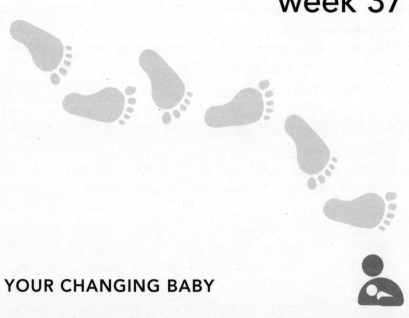

week 37

YOUR CHANGING BABY

You are now considered 'full term'. This means that, although you may be three weeks from your due date, your baby is fully developed and mature and should be able to cope after birth without difficulty. He produces lots of cortisol so that his lungs make surfactant to help with his breathing. All his organs are functioning. His heart still beats much faster than yours – between 110 and 160 beats per minute.

The majority of your baby's lanugo hair, the soft down that covered his body to protect it from the amniotic fluid, has been shed. He may have also lost some of his vernix, the waxy coating on his skin, though some may still be present when he is born. These substances are lost into the amniotic fluid and are swallowed by your baby; they are some of the components that make up the meconium, which will be his first bowel motion.

Your baby's face has filled out due to his weight gain. His facial features are fully developed, including eyelashes and eyebrows. He may even have a full head of hair. He continues to grow and put on weight. As your bump increases in size, the skin over your abdomen becomes stretched and lets in more light and dark, so your baby develops activity cycles – periods of being awake and asleep. The average foetus measures approximately 49 centimetres (1 foot 7 inches) in length and weighs about 2.9 kilograms (6 pounds 6 ounces).

YOUR CHANGING BODY

Your baby may not yet have engaged, especially if this is not your first pregnancy, and may not engage until just before or even during labour. In a first pregnancy, the muscles will be tighter as they have not been stretched. This means that they put more pressure on your baby's head, forcing it down into your pelvis to become engaged. In a second or subsequent pregnancy, the muscles don't exert the same amount of pressure, so your baby's head may not engage until just before labour.

In preparation for labour and delivery, hormones such as relaxin loosen the ligaments and joints in your pelvis further to allow your baby to pass through the birth canal. Relaxin also helps to ripen your cervix, making it softer, shorter and thinner in preparation for dilating during labour.

'I'VE HAD ENOUGH!'

By this point in pregnancy most women have 'had enough', and it is extremely common to feel frustrated and impatient or become irritable. The combination of being tired and heavy with understandable anxieties or concerns about labour can be very wearing. Not knowing when labour will happen can also be frustrating as it is difficult to ready yourself for an event when you don't know when it will occur!

You may have planned everything from childcare for other children and packing your hospital bag to stocking your freezer. Now many women feel they have entered a limbo or waiting phase as they wait for their babies to arrive. Friends and family may start phoning asking if there is any news, or how long there is to go. This can be extremely frustrating, especially when you are having to get up every hour or so during the night to go to the toilet because the baby is pressing on your bladder, and need your partner to help you get out of bed in the morning! Try to remember that there is not long to go before the baby will arrive, even if you do go overdue. If you feel that you are becoming overwhelmed by your emotions or your concerns regarding labour, do talk to your antenatal team.

YOGA

Partial legs-up-the-wall pose

This can be great for swollen ankles and tired legs.

- Lie on your side on the floor with your bottom right next to the wall. Bend your knees into your chest (as much as you can without putting pressure on your bump).
- Turn as if you were going to lie on your back, but place a small pillow or block under your lower back so that you are lying slightly on your side.
- Lift your top leg up the wall. Breathe. Bring your leg down.
- Bring your knees up to your chest and roll to your other side to repeat with the second leg.
- To come out of the pose, bring your leg down, your knees up to your chest and roll on to your side before coming up on your hands and knees to stand up.

'The waiting is so frustrating. I feel heavy and tired, but more than that I feel ready. I have everything we need and am ready and waiting for the baby. I just want to meet it – soon!' Marina, 29

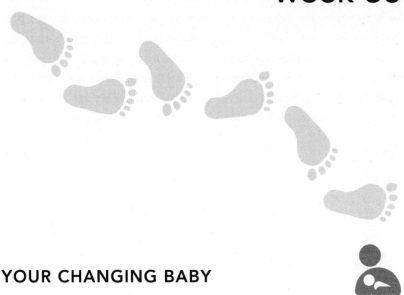

week 38

YOUR CHANGING BABY

Your baby is fully developed and is in the position in which he will be born, though he will continue to put on weight while he is inside your womb. The majority of the lanugo hair has been shed but you may notice he still has a bit remaining when he is born, which will disappear on its own. Most of the vernix has also disappeared but some remains to help his passage during labour as it makes his skin moist and slippery.

All his organs are functioning and he continues to practise the movements required for breathing and swallowing. In boys, the testicles have descended into the scrotum, and in girls the breasts may be slightly swollen due to the effect of your hormones – these will return to normal soon after birth. Your placenta is fully mature and weighs approximately 700 grams (1 pound 9 ounces). The average foetus measures approximately 50 centimetres (1 foot 7½ inches) in length and weighs about 3 kilograms (6 pounds 10 ounces).

YOUR CHANGING BODY

You probably will have noticed an increase in your vaginal discharge during your pregnancy, though this should have been clear or white in colour and non-offensive in smell. During the last few weeks of pregnancy the amount of discharge may increase even further and you may have to use a panty liner. You might notice that the

'MY BABY IS MOVING LESS THAN BEFORE. IS HE OKAY?'

It is quite common to notice that your baby's movements feel different in the last few weeks of pregnancy because there is less room for him to move around. However, although the quality of the movements may change, the quantity should be the same – you should still feel movements regularly. If you are concerned that you have not felt any foetal movements, or there are fewer movements than normal, try to encourage your baby to move by changing position, lying down, giving your bump a tap, poke or prod or even coughing. Often you will feel your baby move in response. If you continue not to feel any movements, if there has been a significant change in the movements or if you are concerned then you should go to your local hospital for assessment. They will listen to the baby's heartbeat using a cardiotocograph (CTG) for a period of about 30 minutes.

discharge turns a light pink colour, especially if you have had sexual intercourse. This is because your cervix is softening in preparation for labour and can bleed slightly when it is touched, such as during sex. However, unless you are specifically told otherwise by your antenatal team, sex is still safe at this late stage of pregnancy. If you are unsure about whether or not your discharge is normal inform your antenatal team, and if you have any bleeding you will need to be assessed urgently by your doctors.

ANTENATAL APPOINTMENT

As with all your appointments you will be examined, your blood pressure taken and your urine tested. If you have any concerns then inform your midwife or doctor. Your team may reiterate the signs of active labour. They may also discuss your options if the baby goes overdue (see Week 40).

STOCKING THE FREEZER

Once you come home with your baby you will probably find that you are extremely busy looking after him and trying to get some sleep. You are likely to have less time for other things so it can be useful to plan for this by stocking up on household essentials. Consider stocking your freezer with healthy meals that you can just take out, defrost and reheat so you don't have to worry about what to feed the family.

Freezing meals in advance does not necessarily mean using bought ready meals – these are often high in both fat and salt content. Instead, you can cheaply prepare large amounts of food, divide it up into portion sizes and then freeze them. Foods that freeze well include:

- soups – you could try vegetable, minestrone, squash or bean
- shepherd's pie
- spaghetti Bolognese
- lasagne
- chicken, beef or fish pie
- casseroles
- stews
- curries

You could even portion up chicken pieces, steaks or lamb chops and freeze them in small bags or containers with the components of a marinade in which the meat will soak as it defrosts prior to cooking. A little preparation may give you a lot of peace of mind!

'She is a bit uncomfortable now and needs help getting up off the sofa, which she hates. She says she feels fat and ugly and says she wants it over with, but I have to admit I am a bit scared of her going into labour. I think I'll find it hard watching her in pain. She tells me not to be a coward and says if I pass out, she won't be happy!'
Mick, 28

week 39

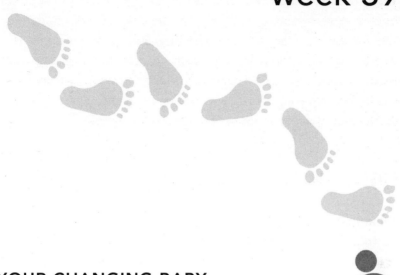

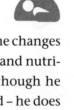

YOUR CHANGING BABY

Although your baby is ready for birth there will still be some changes in his body after he is born. Currently he gets his oxygen and nutritional requirements from you, via the placenta, and although he practises breathing – inhaling and exhaling amniotic fluid – he does not use his lungs for oxygen transfer as they are filled with water. Once he is born he will need to send blood to his lungs to get oxygen for use in the rest of his body. As he takes his first breath, the umbilical cord will stop working and various and quite complex changes will be made in his heart and circulatory system to allow this to happen. This generally occurs without the need for any help, though it might take a few hours for his breathing pattern to become normal.

Only 3 per cent of babies are breech by this point in pregnancy. The majority of babies are head down with their arms and legs pulled into their chests, the so-called 'foetal position', ready for their passage through the birth canal. The average foetus measures approximately 51 centimetres (1 foot 8 inches) in length and weighs about 3.3–3.4 kilograms (7 pounds 6 ounces).

YOUR CHANGING BODY

Your breasts are ready for breastfeeding. Some women notice that they are already producing colostrum – a clear fluid – or even milk. Your breasts will increase in size and feel full. Don't worry if you don't leak any fluid; your breasts will still be ready and will respond to delivery and your baby's suckling by producing milk.

SIGNS OF LABOUR STARTING

A common concern women have as they approach the end of their pregnancy is being able to recognise when labour is starting. Do not worry if you go into hospital for what turns out to be a 'false alarm'. These are very common as it can be difficult to know what to expect from labour, especially if this is your first time.

The 'show'

During pregnancy there is a thick plug of mucus in your cervical canal to prevent an infection, or any other substances, getting into the sterile environment of your womb. This plug has to be lost before the baby can be delivered. During the last few weeks and days of pregnancy your cervix changes and ripens ready for labour. Ordinarily, your cervix is long and firm; now it becomes soft and shortens so that it can dilate or widen to allow passage of your baby through the birth canal.

As the cervix ripens, the mucus plug can be dislodged and is seen as a 'show', which women may notice as a blob of mucus in their knickers. The show can sometimes look bloody as there may be a small amount of bleeding from your cervix, which is normal. If you are concerned then go to your labour ward or maternity unit for assessment. The show does not always mean that labour is just about to start, but hopefully indicates that it will start soon!

Contractions

Your Braxton Hicks contractions may occur more frequently and feel stronger in intensity in the lead-up to labour. However, these practice contractions are generally still irregular. When labour truly starts the contractions will become regular and will increase in intensity.

You may notice that you are having regular contractions but that they are quite widely spaced, say every 30 minutes or so. If this is your first baby you may notice these irregular contractions earlier; if you have had a baby before, your womb will be more efficient at contracting this time. In established labour you will have contractions, felt in your lower abdomen or back, at least every 15 minutes or so, increasing in frequency, strength, intensity and length. You can time the contractions, from the time one starts until the next one starts. For example, if a contraction lasts 30 seconds and then there is a gap of 9 minutes and 30 seconds until the next one starts, the contractions are 10 minutes apart (for more information on contractions, or for when to go to hospital, see page 249).

'I spent the first three months of my pregnancy worrying that every twinge or ache I felt in my tummy meant that something was going wrong. Now I think that every twinge means I am going into labour! I keep getting two or three contractions and then nothing for hours.' Jennifer, 31

Waters breaking

You may notice that you have a gush of clear fluid from below, or that your vaginal discharge becomes profuse and watery. This could be because your membranes have ruptured (your waters have broken), though it can be difficult to distinguish a small amount of fluid from urine.

If you think your waters have broken you will need to go into hospital for assessment, even if you are not having contractions. Labour generally starts soon after the membranes rupture, but if it does not there is a risk of infection to the baby so you may be started on antibiotics. If you show any signs of infection, labour may be induced. It is also common for your waters not to break until labour has progressed significantly further, or for a midwife to break your waters for you when you are in hospital.

If you are experiencing regular contractions, your waters have broken or you are concerned in any way you should contact your labour ward, which will have staff available 24 hours a day, seven days a week. Depending on your medical and obstetric history, they may advise you to stay at home until the contractions become more frequent and regular, perhaps having a warm bath to help with the pain in the meantime. If you are anxious or concerned then you can always go down to your local unit to be assessed.

What happens when you get to hospital?

When you get to the hospital your blood pressure and other vital signs will be checked. The baby's heart rate may be monitored for a short period using a cardiotocograph (for more information see 'Monitoring during Labour', page 254). If your contractions are occurring regularly and your cervix has dilated to approximately 3–4 centimetres you will be in true labour. If your contractions have slowed down or your cervix is not dilated you may be in the early stages of labour. You may be advised to go home until the contractions start again or you may be allowed to stay on the antenatal ward if you have other medical concerns or are extremely anxious.

YOGA

Yoga can be performed throughout pregnancy, even into the last few weeks. The following two stretches may help with backache.

Standing side stretch

- Stand with feet 2–3 feet apart, toes turned slightly outwards, knees slightly bent.
- Bend the upper body to one side and rest that hand or arm on the thigh.
- Then inhale and lift the opposite arm up and stretch it over your head.
- Hold for five deep breaths before straightening up.

Sitting side stretch and twist

- Sit up straight with your legs crossed in front of you.
- As you inhale, lift your right arm straight up so your fingers are pointing towards the ceiling.
- As you exhale, put your left arm with your fingertips (or palm if you can) on the floor directly next to your hip.
- Keep breathing and, with your right arm, reach up and over your head, stretching over to your left side, keeping your right hip firmly anchored to the floor. Breathe into this stretch, which helps to open the waist.

- Inhale and straighten up, with your right arm straight up to the ceiling.
- Place your right hand on to your left knee and twist to look over your left shoulder. Breathe. When twisting, think of turning your spine above your bump to help loosen the middle and upper spine.
- Come back to the centre and repeat on the other side.

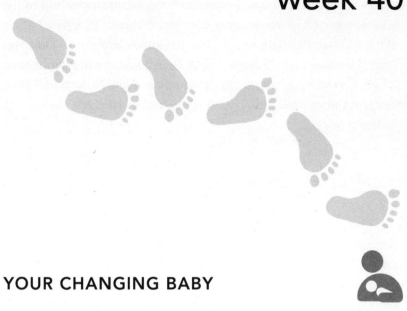

week 40

YOUR CHANGING BABY

Your baby's organs are functioning and he is ready to be born: his kidneys are producing urine; his liver is working; his gut is full of meconium for his first bowel motion. He can move and control his arms and legs; he can see, smell, hear, touch and taste, and has various newborn reflexes. As much as his brain has developed in the past nine months it will continue to grow and new connections will be made as he grows and learns over the next months and years.

He will continue to be active, squirming and moving from side to side or kicking to get comfortable. The bones of his head are still soft and pliable; they will slide over each other to decrease the size of his head so that he can pass through the birth canal. Although the placenta begins to age, it still supplies your baby with all his oxygen and nutritional requirements.

There is a theory that the baby himself triggers labour when ready, by stimulating the production of the hormones required to contract the uterus. At birth, the average foetus measures approximately 50–51 centimetres (1 foot 8 inches) in length and weighs about 3.5 kilograms (7 pounds 11 ounces). Boys tend to weigh slightly more than girls. The diameter of his head will be about 10 centimetres (4 inches), and the average umbilical cord is approximately 55–60 centimetres (1 foot 10 inches) in length. These are only average measurements; your baby's length and weight will be dependent on various factors including the parents' height and ethnicity, and whether you are a smoker or have diabetes. Weights can range between approximately 2.5 and 4.5 kilograms (5 pounds 8 ounces to 9 pounds 14 ounces), though can be even smaller or larger.

YOUR CHANGING BODY

Your body has changed dramatically from its pre-pregnancy state, adapting to meet the needs of your growing baby and preparing for labour. Every system in your body has been affected. You have produced more blood and your heart is working harder than previously. Your internal organs have shifted to accommodate your hugely expanded womb, and your breasts are now ready for breastfeeding. Not only has your appearance changed, but you will also have already begun the bonding process with your baby and started to prepare for labour and life with a baby. These changes have taken nine months, but after delivery your body will return to its pre-pregnancy state in approximately six weeks.

'IS THERE ANYTHING I CAN DO TO HELP START LABOUR?'

Many women are keen for labour to start by the time they reach the 40th week of pregnancy. There are various natural 'remedies' that may help to kick-start labour, though none is proven or infallible! Many women report that eating spicy foods such as curry (if they do not normally eat them) or drinking raspberry leaf tea can start labour. Movements such as climbing the stairs sideways in a crab-like action may help as it rocks the baby's head down on to the cervix; even walking may help. Perhaps one of the best-known methods is sexual intercourse – semen contains prostaglandins which can help to ripen the cervix, and the hormone released at orgasm is the same as that which induces contractions, though sex will only start labour if it was about to start anyway. Stimulating the nipples can also help to release oxytocin to stimulate contractions.

ANTENATAL APPOINTMENT

If this is your first pregnancy you will be offered an antenatal appointment at 40 weeks. This will follow the same structure as your previous appointments, and further discussions may be had regarding labour, what will happen if you go overdue and life after the birth. A further antenatal appointment will be arranged at 41 weeks, if you have not delivered your baby, whether or not this is your first pregnancy.

BREATHING TECHNIQUES FOR LABOUR

As a normal reaction to pain your breathing becomes very shallow and fast. This means that you are not using your breathing effectively and can even overbreathe or hyperventilate. One method for trying to stay relaxed during labour is to focus on your breathing. If you have been practising yogic breathing (see page 71) you can continue to use this; if not you may like to practise some breathing techniques for use in labour. Focus on your breathing and try to keep it slow and regular. You may like to inhale to a count of three, and then exhale in the same way. Focus on the out-breath or exhalation and try to make it slightly longer than your in-breath; some women find this easier if they breathe in through the nose and out through the mouth. You could recite a two-syllable word in your head as you breathe – the first syllable as you inhale, the second as

YOGA POSE FOR LABOUR

The yogic squat pose can be used throughout labour, even during the pushing stage.

- Start with your feet slightly wider than hip-width apart and turn your toes slightly outwards.
- Take a breath in and, as you exhale, hold on to something solid, such as a window ledge or towel rail. Gradually lower your bottom towards the floor, all the way down, squatting as deeply as you can while keeping your heels on the floor. You might like to use a block, rolled towel or pillow for support under your bottom and to help take some of the weight off your feet.
- Bring your hands together in front of your chest in a prayer position. Your elbows can rest by your knees, gently pushing them back. You might like to ask your partner to help support you in this position.
- To come up, lean forwards and place your hands shoulder-width apart on the floor, then go on to all fours before pushing back on to the feet and standing up.

you exhale – such as 'relax', 'quiet' or 'baby'. You could also try the joined breathing described in Week 12. Your partner can help you control your breathing by counting your inhalations and exhalations for you.

Some women find it helpful to simulate contractions by pinching themselves or touching their arm or leg with an ice cube and then practising their breathing at the same time – though of course don't hurt yourself! In labour there may also be times when you will be asked to try not to push; here you can use your breathing to help you by using a short panting technique. It can be helpful to practise these breathing techniques so you will be comfortable using them during labour.

OVERDUE BABIES

Babies are considered full term if they are born between 37 and 42 weeks' gestation. Only approximately 5 per cent of babies are born on their expected delivery date, with about 25 per cent being born earlier and 70 per cent being delivered later than the EDD. Of those women who have not delivered by their due date, the majority will deliver in the 40th week, with a few going into the 41st week. It is not recommended that babies be allowed to stay in the womb beyond 42 weeks as the placenta begins to age and stops functioning so well.

If you have not delivered by Week 41 you will be offered an antenatal appointment where your doctor will examine you vaginally and assess how 'ripe' your cervix is – its length, firmness and whether or not there is any dilation. If possible, the doctor may carry out a vaginal 'sweep'. This involves inserting a finger into the cervix to sweep the amniotic membranes, which contain the baby and amniotic fluid, away from the cervix. This action releases prostaglandins, a chemical which may start contractions. The procedure itself may be slightly uncomfortable but should not be painful.

If a sweep is not possible because your cervix is too tightly closed, or if the sweep is not effective, you will probably be booked in for an induction of labour at some point during your 41st week. This gives you more time to go into labour on your own, without letting you go over 42 weeks' gestation. At some point during your wait you will be asked to come in, generally to the maternity day unit or antenatal ward, so that your baby can be assessed using a cardiotocograph to check that there are no problems. You may also be offered an ultrasound scan. (For more information on monitoring the baby see page 255.)

Induction of labour

Induction of labour is used to kick-start labour in various circumstances. It may be used, for example, for the safety of the foetus, if there are concerns such as reduced growth, or if the amniotic membranes have broken and there are concerns about infection. Perhaps the most common foetal reason for induction of labour is postmaturity – when pregnancy has gone on into the 41st week. Labour may be induced for the safety of the mother, such as in cases of severe pre-eclampsia (for more information see page 155).

How labour is induced will depend on whether or not you have had a baby previously and how 'ripe' your cervix is, as a cervical sweep (see above) may be enough to start labour. This may be offered to you at an antenatal appointment. If the sweep does not start labour, you will be induced using medication unless there are contraindications such as a previous Caesarean section. How 'ripe' or favourable your cervix is for induction is measured using the Bishop's score. When your doctor or midwife examines you they will assess various factors such as whether or not you are dilated at all, and how firm or soft your cervix is. The higher your score, the more likely it is that induction will be successful.

For an induction of labour you will be asked to come into the antenatal ward, usually at night if this is your first baby, or in the morning if you have previously had a baby. Your baby will be monitored using a cardiotocograph, generally on admission and then after every medication or procedure. You will be offered a vaginal pessary or gel of prostaglandin, the same chemical that is produced naturally in the body. The prostaglandin helps to ripen the cervix. You can be given doses every six hours, although in some units only one dose of a slow-releasing prostaglandin is given which can last 24 hours. Women who have not had a baby previously often need an extra dose, or doses, of prostaglandin; they are asked to come in at night as labour probably won't start until the next morning.

If your cervix starts to change and dilate, it may be possible to artificially rupture your membranes (break your waters) once it reaches approximately 2–3 centimetres. Your doctor or midwife will examine you and use a small instrument to rupture your membranes through your cervix. The examination may be a bit uncomfortable but is generally very quick and followed by a gush of fluid as your waters come out. Often, this may be enough to trigger labour.

If labour hasn't yet started after the pessary, or it is not possible to rupture your membranes, or if rupture does not trigger contractions, you may be advised to go on a drip of syntocinon. This is an artificial form of the hormone oxytocin, which is naturally produced in the brain. Your uterus has been developing lots of receptors for oxytocin during your pregnancy, which will make your womb contract. While the medication is being delivered through a drip, your baby will be constantly monitored with a cardiotocograph. A risk of syntocinon is that it makes the uterus contract too much. If this occurs the syntocinon will be slowed or stopped and, if required, a medication given to relax the uterus and stop the contractions.

More women request an epidural during an induced labour, and many report that the contractions of an induced labour are more painful than in natural labour. However, there are lots of options for pain relief.

Artificially induced labours can seem longer than those that occur naturally. This is probably not the case if you include the slow or latent phase of labour (see page 246). This can take many hours or even a day or so in natural labour, where very irregular and mild contractions occur and the cervix ripens and changes.

There is also a risk that the induction fails – that your cervix does not dilate, or that it dilates to a point but no further. In this case, or earlier if the baby is becoming stressed or compromised, you may be advised to have a Caesarean section.

The list of potential disadvantages or side-effects of an induced labour appears long, but these have to be weighed up against the risks of continuing a pregnancy where you or the baby may be at risk, so induction can be favourable. Although it may not be what you had planned or hoped for, your labour can still go smoothly and be a good experience.

'Okay, I'm ready. The freezer is full, my bag is packed, including snacks for my husband. All the contact numbers are in my phone, my car, my handbag and on the fridge. I have plans for my son for every day for the next week or so and plans if it happens at night. Everyone is on high alert – bring it on!' Zoë, 30

labour

The birth of a baby is a miraculous and wondrous event, but at the same time it is painful, tiring and messy. It can make you feel powerful as a woman, or even quite humble and scared that you now actually have a real live baby!

There is a lot of pressure aimed at women regarding natural delivery, avoiding pain relief and their labour becoming 'medicalised'. Remember, though, that the aim of care during labour is to ensure the health of both you and your baby. Keep an open mind: every labour in every woman is different, and you and your team of carers will together choose the best options for you and your baby.

WHAT TRIGGERS LABOUR?

We don't know exactly what triggers labour or why it occurs earlier or later in some women than in others. There are various theories: one proposes that the levels of the hormone oxytocin secreted from the woman's brain increase, leading to contractions. Other theories focus on the baby setting off labour when it is mature, perhaps by secreting a hormone from its adrenal glands; this hormone could then cause hormonal changes in the woman to initiate labour. It may be a combination of factors. (For natural methods that may help encourage labour to start see Week 40.)

The length of all the stages of labour will be different in different women, though first labours tend to be the longest. However long it takes, just remember that every contraction is one contraction closer to seeing your baby for the first time.

THE FIRST STAGE

Here we go ... Unlike in films or on television, the first stage of labour can take quite a while. You may not even be aware that it has started, so you probably don't need to panic that the baby will arrive straight after two contractions! The first stage of labour is defined as starting at the onset of regular contractions up until the point when the cervix is fully dilated to 10 centimetres. It may also be referred to as the stage of dilatation. Regular contractions come every five, six, eight or ten minutes, for example, and keep coming for over an hour. Irregular contractions come now and again, so you may get three or four every five minutes and then nothing for an hour or so. You should go to hospital when the contractions are five minutes apart and last a minute each (for more information about when to go to hospital see page 249).

The first stage of labour is the longest and is often subdivided into three stages: the latent phase, the active phase and, in some women, the transition phase.

The latent phase

The latent phase is the first part of the first stage of labour. During this time various changes will be occurring in your cervix. Many women notice some irregular, generally mild contractions, which are often described as similar to the discomfort felt during a period. As with period pain, some women notice the pain or discomfort in their lower abdomen and others in their lower back.

This phase varies in length, from hours to even a few days; it is generally longer in first-time mothers. If you have had a baby previously the latent phase may be much shorter, and as your womb has already had practice at contractions you may not even be aware of anything happening. Many women feel the need to open their bowels during the early stages of labour.

Prior to and throughout your pregnancy your cervix is thick, firm and approximately 2 centimetres long. Hormones such as relaxin, which are secreted during the later weeks of pregnancy, start to soften the cervix. During the latent phase of labour the cervix changes further, becoming softer and thinner and then progressively shorter in length. This process is called effacement of the cervix and needs to occur before the cervix can dilate, or stretch open.

Effacement occurs as the contractions gradually pull the cervix upwards towards (and during the later stages of labour, eventually over) the baby's head or presenting part. These contractions can be difficult to distinguish from Braxton Hicks contractions (see Week 34), in that they are both considered mild and irregular. You may notice that the contractions become more regular during the latent phase, for example occurring three to four times per hour. The latent phase of labour is generally considered to end when the cervix has

'I had hoped that I would be like my friend who felt nothing, and then her contractions started all in one go, she went to the hospital and was already 4 centimetres dilated. Not for me. I had contractions for at least a day before they really got going. One here, three or four in a row there ... With every bout of contractions my husband got all excited that it was really starting. By the time I did get going with regular contractions I think he'd had enough!' Monique, 31

dilated to 4 centimetres and the cervix is fully effaced, at which point the active phase of labour begins.

For some women, particularly first-time mothers, these early contractions are painful. When you are at home you may find that a warm bath or a back rub can help with the discomfort. If the pain is too much for you to deal with at home then contact your labour ward; you may be advised to come into hospital to be offered pain relief (for more information on pain relief see page 260). (See also 'When should I go to hospital?', page 249.)

The active phase

Once the cervix has dilated to 4 centimetres and the contractions become increasingly regular and intense, the active phase of the first stage of labour has started.

The active stage lasts until the cervix is fully dilated, at 10 centimetres. Towards the end of this phase the baby's presenting part (generally the head) drops right down into the cavity of the pelvis in preparation for delivery. The contractions continue, becoming more regular and stronger in intensity. They start at the top, or fundus, of the uterus and spread downwards to push the baby's head against your cervix to stretch or dilate it. The contractions will become increasingly painful and are generally felt in the centre or all over your bump, as if a band is being tightened across it; some women report that they feel them most in their lower back. If you touch your bump you can feel the uterus becoming hard during a contraction.

The pain of contractions is due to chemicals released by the muscle cells in the wall of your womb; these chemicals are released when blood supply to the cells is temporarily cut off during contractions (as the blood vessels are squeezed). As the contraction subsides these chemicals are removed, so you have a recovery period between contractions. At the end of pregnancy your uterus is large and powerful, and so can produce strong, and therefore painful, contractions (for information about methods of pain relief see page 260).

'WHEN SHOULD I GO TO HOSPITAL?'

There is no hard and fast rule as to when to go to
your labour ward or birthing unit. It depends on
various factors, such as the distance between your
home and the hospital, and how you are feeling or
managing any pain or discomfort. You may be
advised to go in early if, for example, you previously
had a very quick labour. If you are coping okay, then
contact your labour ward to tell them how often the
contractions are coming and how long they are
lasting and they will advise you. To time contractions,
start at the beginning of one contraction and time
how long it lasts, then note the time between the
beginning of one contraction and the beginning of
the next. If your contractions are coming every five
minutes and lasting for approximately a minute, and
have done so for about an hour, it is probably time to
go to hospital.

The contractions continue to increase in frequency and intensity and
are timed from the beginning of one contraction to the start of the
next. Although contractions may initially have been every 15
minutes, as the active phase progresses they may occur every 5
minutes, or every 2 minutes. The contractions also increase in length,
lasting between a minute and a minute and a half, though you could
think of each contraction rising gradually to a peak before fading
away. If your contractions are coming every two to three minutes the

recovery period can be brief, though remember that every contraction brings delivery one step closer.

The active phase of the first stage of labour can last a varying amount of time. For first pregnancies, the cervix will dilate at the rate of approximately 1 centimetre per hour, though in subsequent pregnancies it may dilate at a faster rate. If your progress is significantly slower than this due to inefficient contractions, you may be offered a drip of syntocinon to help speed up your contractions, or an artificial rupture of membranes (for more information see page 243). Labour may also be slow or prolonged if the baby does not descend into the pelvis (for example if the baby is very big and the pelvis is small) or turn into the best position for delivery. In most cases, prolonged labour is due to a combination of the above.

> 'By the end of the first stage I was getting quite tired. The contractions were coming so fast it almost felt like there wasn't a break in between them. But it wasn't like period pain or a headache. I really felt my pain had a purpose, which helped me cope with it. Each pain helped me to bring my baby out.' Verity, 28

The transition phase

The transition phase does not always occur, though if it does it can last from a few minutes to an hour. It can be thought of as a pause between the dilation of the cervix in the active phase and the pushing stage of the second stage of labour. The contractions continue and can be intense, but as yet you may not feel an urge to push. Some women have the urge to push before they are fully dilated. If you feel you want to push tell your midwife who will examine you first; if you are not fully dilated you will be encouraged to try not to push by taking short panting breaths during your contractions.

It is important not to push too early as the cervix will not be dilated enough to allow the baby's head to pass through it, and the pushing can cause problems for you later in life such as increasing the risk of urinary incontinence. Some women find that the urge to push decreases if they change position to ease the pressure of the baby's head on the cervix, such as moving on to their hands and knees or over a birthing ball.

'When will my waters break?'

In the majority of cases, approximately 85 per cent of women, labour starts before the membranes surrounding the placenta, baby and amniotic fluid rupture and the 'waters break'. This means that in approximately 15 per cent of women the waters break before labour; in most of these cases labour starts soon afterwards, generally within the next 24 hours. If your waters break you need to go to hospital as if contractions do not start there is a risk of infection. Women are generally started on antibiotics after 18 hours if contractions do not start. Depending on your particular circumstances and whether or not you are at term, your doctors may recommend that labour is induced.

If your membranes do not spontaneously rupture before labour starts, you will probably find that your waters break during labour. If your labour is progressing slowly, or if you have been induced, you

'I had images of my waters breaking like they do in films, with me standing on a bus and drenching my shoes and everyone else around me. It wasn't quite like that. I was in the hospital and felt wet down below. A few minutes later the midwife changed the pads I was sitting on and we were one step closer to having a baby.' Vanessa, 25

POSITIONS FOR THE FIRST STAGE

The first stage can take many hours, so it is likely that you will change position a few times. Many women spend some time in a warm bath, walking or trying to rest. Positions you might like to try include:

- Sitting – try sitting facing the back of the chair, leaning on it with your arms for support. Your partner could rub your lower back.
- Supported sitting – your partner sits behind you (supporting himself against the back of the bed or a wall) and you sit in between his legs in front of him, leaning back for support.
- Leaning – you stand and face your partner with your arms around him, leaning forward so that he is supporting some of your weight. Again, this may be a good position for a back massage.
- Walking – you may find moving and walking helpful during the first stage. In between contractions you may like to rest by leaning on your partner or the back of a chair.
- Birthing ball – these are very large, air-filled plastic balls which can be used in a variety of positions to support you during labour. Your labour ward may have birthing balls or you may be advised to bring your own.

may be offered an artificial rupture of membranes – or amniotomy. This is because rupturing the membranes releases chemicals called prostaglandins that help increase the rate of contractions. Rupturing the membranes, be it spontaneously or artificially, also puts more pressure from the baby's head on to the cervix, as the cushioning effect from the amniotic fluid is removed.

In some hospitals, all women are offered artificial rupture of membranes if the waters have not broken by the time their cervix is dilated to approximately 5 centimetres, though as long as everything is progressing naturally this is not a necessity. It is done with the aim of speeding up labour, though some women prefer to have no intervention unless absolutely necessary. You may like to ask about your obstetric unit's policy regarding artificial rupture of membranes prior to your labour, or you could include your views about it on your birth plan (for more information about artificial rupture of membranes see Week 40).

'Is it safe to eat and drink in labour?'

If everything is going well it is considered safe to eat and drink, even when you are in established labour. Although you probably won't want a three-course meal, labour can be hungry and thirsty work. You may like to eat lightly but quite often, choosing snacks such as bananas, toast or cereal. These are better choices than sugary snacks as they are slow-releasing high-energy foods. You should keep drinking during your labour, again little and often. The National Institute of Clinical Excellence currently recommends that drinking isotonic drinks, like those given to athletes, may be better than drinking water as they replace both fluid and salts in the body.

If you have been given pethidine, have had an epidural or become likely to need a Caesarean, you will be advised not to eat (just in case, in rare circumstances, you have to have a general anaesthetic it is safer to have an empty stomach), but depending on the exact circumstances you may still be allowed to have drinks. If you are likely to have a Caesarean you may be offered some ranitidine, a medication to stop your stomach producing acid. Different units may have different policies regarding eating and drinking in labour, so do ask. After it's all over, you will probably be offered a well-deserved cup of tea and some toast!

MONITORING DURING LABOUR

Monitoring you

How often you are examined during labour will depend on your particular set of circumstances. In general, women are examined on admission to hospital, to check that the cervix has dilated and that labour has actually started. Thereafter, if there are no concerns you will be examined every four hours during the active phase of the first stage. You will also be examined when you say that you feel the urge to push, in order to check that your cervix is fully dilated to 10 centimetres. If there are any concerns, you may be examined more regularly.

The midwife will generally examine first your bump to feel the baby's lie and presentation, that is whether she can feel your baby's head or his bottom (or foot), and then examine you vaginally to examine your cervix to see that it is dilating at the appropriate rate. If the baby is head down, the midwife then checks whether the baby's face is facing your spine so the back of his head is facing your tummy (occipito-anterior position or OA), or if his face is facing your tummy so his spine is facing your spine (occipito-posterior or OP), or facing the side (occipito-transverse or OT). Labours where the baby's head is OP are often longer as a wider part of the baby's head is presenting first. The best presentation for delivery is OA, though the baby may start in a different presentation, such as OT, during early labour and rotate before delivery.

Your midwife will also check how far the baby's head or presenting part has descended into the pelvis. This is called the station: if baby's head can be felt at the narrowest part of your pelvis (at a point called the ischial spines) the station is zero. Your midwife measures (using her fingers) how far above or below this point your baby's head can be felt. These measurements are in centimetres; negative numbers are used if the head is above the ischial spines, positive numbers if it is below. So, you can be 10 centimetres, or fully, dilated and the station may be zero; as you start pushing the station will become positive as the baby's head gets lower and your baby closer to being born.

Monitoring the baby

The muscles of the uterus contract during contractions, and blood vessels that run in this muscle to supply the placenta are compressed. This means that, during a contraction, the oxygen supply to the foetus temporarily decreases. This is generally shown by a slowing in the foetal heart rate at the peak of contractions. Some babies become stressed during labour, for various reasons, such as not receiving enough oxygen. This can be picked up by examining changes in the pattern and speed of their heartbeats, which is why babies are monitored during labour.

Various methods can be used to monitor the baby. The aim of foetal monitoring is to ensure that the baby is coping with the stresses of labour, and that the midwife and, if necessary, the medical team are aware if the baby has become compromised and needs to be delivered quickly. If you have had an uncomplicated pregnancy and your labour is progressing well the monitoring can be done intermittently, though if there are any concerns then continuous monitoring may be advised (see overleaf).

Pinard's stethoscope or Doppler sonicaid
A Pinard's stethoscope is a method of listening to the baby's heartbeat. A stethoscope shaped like a trumpet is placed on your bump and the midwife puts her ear on the other side. A Doppler sonicaid is a machine that uses ultrasound waves to detect the baby's heartbeat, and is often used both in antenatal appointments and during labour. Waterproof sonicaids are available for use in water births.

Generally, the midwife will listen to the baby's heartbeat regularly, every 15 minutes during the first stage of labour. In the second stage, the pushing stage, the foetus's heartbeat will be examined after every contraction.

Electronic foetal monitoring

Electronic foetal monitoring can be performed externally with a cardiotocograph (CTG) or internally using foetal scalp electrodes. A CTG is a machine that monitors both your baby's heart rate and your contractions continuously. It uses two small pads or sensors strapped to your abdomen and attached to the machine by a lead, so you cannot move far from the machine. The CTG gives a printout of the pattern and rate of the heartbeat as well as the pattern of your contractions, and the foetal heartbeat can also be heard.

Internal foetal monitoring is used if it is difficult to pick up the baby's heartbeat externally, or if other forms of monitoring show changes in the baby's heart rate and it is necessary to know its heart beat accurately. Here, you are examined vaginally and a small electrode is clipped to the baby's head to pick up its heartbeat; a sensor is strapped to your bump to monitor your contractions. The electrode or clip may leave a small mark or scratch on the baby's head which should heal within a few days of delivery. This all sounds quite scary but in fact monitoring often gives women reassurance that the baby is carefully being watched.

Electronic foetal monitoring can be used continuously or intermittently as described above for the other monitoring methods. In a healthy pregnancy and labour, continuous foetal monitoring during labour is not necessary. However, you may be advised to have continuous foetal monitoring for various reasons. These include:

- if you were unwell during pregnancy, for example with pre-eclampsia
- if you have an epidural
- if you are carrying a multiple pregnancy (here more sensors are used so each baby's heart rate is monitored separately)

- if there has been bleeding
- if labour has been induced
- if the baby is in a breech presentation

Alternatively, if your midwife has been listening to the heartbeat intermittently and has concerns about the baby's heart rate, you may be advised to have continuous monitoring so any changes will be picked up quickly and acted on if necessary.

The obvious drawback of continuous electronic foetal monitoring is that you are bound by the length of the wires attaching you to the machine. In general, these wires are long enough to let you stand up and move around, change positions or use a birthing ball, though you won't be able to leave your room and stay attached. It is not possible to use the machines and have a water birth. However, a CTG is a good way of monitoring the baby; it is safe and involves only a few pads and wires, so is not invasive.

Foetal blood sampling

In this procedure a tiny sample of the foetus's blood is removed and tested. It is carried out if other methods of monitoring show suspicious changes in the baby's heart rate, or if these other methods are not giving clear results. During a vaginal examination, a device is used to scratch the baby's head to obtain the sample. You will be asked to lie on your side or on your back with your legs raised in stirrups. The blood is then analysed and various measurements are taken, such as the pH (how acid or alkaline the sample is) and bicarbonate levels. If the blood is very acidic it is likely that the baby is not receiving enough oxygen and will need to be delivered. How it is delivered will depend on how far labour has progressed (see overleaf).

What happens if the baby's heart rate changes?

Depending on the results of the foetal monitoring and/or the blood sampling, your midwifery and medical team will discuss the options with you. If the baby is fine, your labour will continue. It may be that the baby does not need delivering immediately but the medical team will keep a close eye on the situation in case things change.

If the baby does need delivering quickly, the way in which it is delivered will depend on how dilated you are and how far the baby has descended into the pelvis. If you are only a few centimetres dilated, a Caesarean may be the only option to deliver the baby quickly. If, however, you are fully dilated and the baby is well descended, an assisted delivery with a ventouse or forceps may be quicker and more appropriate.

It can be upsetting when your birth plan, or idea of how your baby is going to be delivered, has to change. Most women do not envisage that their baby will need urgent delivery. However, your midwifery and medical teams will discuss intervention with you only if it is appropriate and needed for the safety of either your or your baby's health (for more information about assisted deliveries including Caesarean sections see pages 285–290).

If, at any point, your midwife has concerns about the health of either yourself or your baby they will call other members of the obstetric team – other midwives and doctors – to help. Remember, the aim of all your care in pregnancy is to ensure a safe pregnancy, safe delivery and a healthy child. Monitoring helps your midwives and doctors, as well as yourself, make decisions regarding the safety of you and your baby. Keep in mind that although labour is a natural process, some babies need a little help finding their way out into the world.

'I was happy to have any monitoring they suggested. As far as I was concerned, the only thing that mattered was that they kept me and my baby safe, so to be attached to a machine by some wires was hardly a big deal – it's not like I was really going anywhere anyway!'
Alice, 30

'WHY HAVE MY WATERS TURNED DARK GREEN?'

During some labours, your midwife may tell you that there is some meconium in your waters, that is, that they have turned from being clear in colour to yellow or green. The meconium is the medical term for your baby's first stool. Occasionally this is passed during labour, either because your baby is post-term (after 40 weeks) or as a response to foetal stress. If it is seen your midwife will closely monitor your baby's heartbeat and your progress.

FOR FATHERS (FIRST STAGE)

Different women will want or need different things from their partner during labour. Try to discuss what she feels she might want you to do during the first stage. Is she happy for you to be the strong silent type, perhaps just holding her hand or stroking her hair? Or does she want you to be more active, helping her with her breathing techniques or giving her a back rub? Does she respond to gentle verbal encouragement or does she want you to try and talk about other topics altogether? Or does she want you to be the person yelling as loudly as he can for an epidural? Try to remember that it is difficult to plan ahead as to how she may feel or what she may want during labour so be prepared for her to change her mind, and change it quite regularly and rapidly!

The role of the birth partner might be thought of as an advocate for the woman – a person who can communicate her desires and needs if she feels unable to do so. You can also find out information about what is going on and how she is progressing, and you can ask questions for her, such as whether or not she is allowed something to eat or drink, and then go and fetch it for her.

Some men do not feel able to be present during labour. It can be upsetting for them to see their loved one in pain, or they may feel that they would be unable to cope with the situation. Although the woman is the one who is actually giving birth, you will undoubtedly be affected by the process. If you do choose to attend, remember that you are not only present to support your partner to the best of your ability; you are also there for yourself, to have the experience of seeing your child come into the world.

'To be honest I felt quite useless when she was in labour. Once I got her to the birthing unit it was all really up to her, and I felt quite bad watching her in pain, thinking that I was to blame – after all, I got her pregnant! She kept changing her mind – one minute wanting to follow our birth plan, the next yelling at me to get her an epidural. All I could really do was hold her hand (even though she could squeeze pretty hard and got cross if I complained!) and be there for her as best as I could, and afterwards she told me how glad she was I was there. To be honest, I was glad too.' Jonathan, 33

PAIN RELIEF IN LABOUR

The issue of pain relief during labour is and has been a contentious one, with lots of pressure applied to women to go through childbirth naturally. The pressure can be so great that some women even feel that they have somehow 'failed' if they need pain relief or analgesia.

Pain is subjective, which means that no one can tell you how bad your pain is as no one else is feeling it. Different women have different pain thresholds and ability to cope with pain, and there is no denying that childbirth is a painful experience, albeit one with a wonderful outcome. So, try to keep an open mind as you may change your opinion about analgesia as your labour continues. Inform yourself about all the various options so that you can choose what is best and right for you and your baby at the time.

There are two main types of medical pain relief for labour:

- analgesic drugs, which prevent the brain from receiving messages of pain from the body
- regional anaesthesia, where there is a blockage of pain sensation to a specific area using local anaesthetics

Gas and air (Entonox)

Gas and air is a form of pain relief that is inhaled. The gas is a mix of air and nitrous oxide, which is also known as laughing gas. Entonox dulls the sensation of pain and can make you feel light-headed, or as if you are slightly removed from yourself, while using it, but it does not cause significant sedation.

You administer the gas and air yourself by breathing in through a tube containing the mixture. It takes a few seconds to work so start inhaling the Entonox as soon as a contraction starts. Breathe deeply and normally, inhaling and exhaling, not holding your breath. After a few breaths you should find the medication starts to work and the pain begins to lessen. This also helps you to concentrate on your breathing during contractions. Stop using the Entonox as the contraction subsides and then start again at the onset of the next one.

The gas mixture is quickly removed from the body and does not have any long-term effects on either you or the baby. Some women find that the gas and air makes them feel nauseous or vomit, or that they do not like the sensation of disorientation or being out of touch with their surroundings.

261

> 'It took me a while to get the hang of the gas and air. You had to start taking it early in a contraction and then it just made me feel a bit floaty and better able to deal with the pain. Too much, though, and I felt weird and a bit sick, but in the end I got the hang of it.'
> Angharad, 34

Pethidine

Injections of drugs such as pethidine give pain relief to the whole body by blocking the reception of pain signals by the brain. Pethidine is similar to morphine, and is commonly used as analgesia during labour. It belongs to the opioid group of drugs, which can cause drowsiness.

Pethidine is generally given by injection into a large muscle such as your bottom or thigh. It takes approximately 15 minutes to take effect, after which your pain should lessen for a few hours. The injection can then be repeated. The side-effects include nausea and vomiting, drowsiness and sedation. These feelings of drowsiness can make some women feel removed from their body and out of touch with their sensations and emotions. Very occasionally, if the mother is over-sedated she may develop breathing problems.

Pethidine does cross the placenta and can cause sleepiness in the baby, which can affect its heart rate on monitoring. The baby may be so sleepy that he has some difficulties breathing when he is delivered. In the majority of cases the effect wears off, and if required a medication called naloxone can be given to the baby to reverse the effect of the pethidine. However, the advantages of pethidine are that it is a very effective painkiller, which works quickly and can be given by a midwife without the need to wait for an anaesthetist.

Epidural anaesthesia

An epidural involves inserting local anaesthetic into the spinal column and blocks all pain sensation in your bump and below. This can be extremely effective and is used by many women during labour. A small procedure is required to insert the epidural. Although it sounds quite medical, epidurals are done regularly and are performed by an anaesthetist.

You can ask for an epidural whenever you feel you need pain relief, but you may have to wait if the anaesthetist is busy with another woman, and you may be advised against it if you are likely to deliver before the epidural would have a chance to work. Once it is in place, the medications will take effect in 10–30 minutes.

Your blood pressure and pulse will be checked immediately after the epidural is inserted and regularly afterwards. Generally, after an epidural is used, you will be advised to have continuous electronic foetal monitoring with a CTG (see above).

Potential side-effects of epidurals

The sensation in the nerves that supply your bladder may also become blocked so you may not be able to tell if you need the toilet. You may be asked to empty your bladder or your midwife may offer to insert a temporary catheter to drain the urine before the procedure. Depending on your obstetric unit, you may be advised to have a urinary catheter if you have an epidural, though some units will allow you to continue to try and empty your bladder regularly and only insert a catheter if required.

Depending on the dose of local anaesthetic needed, the nerves that supply the motor control to your legs may also become blocked. This may make it difficult or impossible for you to move your legs, which can feel very heavy. Traditional epidurals used high doses of medication, making it likely that women would not be able to move their legs. Modern, mobile epidurals use low doses of anaesthetic drugs to decrease the risk of blocking the motor nerves so you can continue to move around. However, because lower doses of medications are used you may need top-ups of medicine to ensure you stay pain-free.

Some of the nerves involved with the blood vessels in your legs can be affected by the anaesthesia, causing the blood vessels to dilate so blood pools in your legs. This can lead to a drop in your blood pressure, and therefore a decrease in the amount of blood and oxygen going to the placenta and your baby. To prevent this from occurring a drip will be inserted (generally into your hand or arm) and you will be given fluids intravenously. Your blood pressure and pulse will also be monitored regularly.

A minority of women find that they get a headache after an epidural. This is not common and is generally relieved with analgesia or lying flat, but do always tell a midwife or doctor if you get a headache.

HOW IS AN EPIDURAL INSERTED?

- An anaesthetist will perform the epidural after explaining the procedure, answering any questions you may have and asking you to sign a consent form.
- Before the epidural procedure is performed a drip will be inserted into your hand to give fluid directly into your veins. The aim of this is to prevent your blood pressure falling while the epidural is working, which can occur as a side-effect.
- The doctor will use sterile gloves, gowns and equipment to decrease the risk of infection.
- Your lower back will then be cleaned with an antiseptic fluid, which often feels very cold, and some clean covers will be draped over your back.

- You will be asked to lie on your left side with your back to the anaesthetist, bending your knees towards your chest as much as possible. Or you will be asked to sit at the edge of the bed, again with your back to the doctor, and hunch forwards over a pillow, often using a table or your partner for support.
- It is important that you stay extremely still during the procedure. This can be difficult if you are having contractions, so if you do get a contraction, tell the anaesthetist who will stop what s/he is doing for the duration of the contraction.
- The doctor will then feel your back to decide the appropriate point to insert the epidural.
- Using a small needle, some local anaesthetic is then inserted into the skin of your lower back. This can cause a short-lived burning sensation, after which no pain should be felt.
- Once the local anaesthetic has taken effect and you cannot feel any pain, a fine needle is inserted through the bones of your back into the epidural space. You may feel some pressure but not pain at this point. Some women report feeling a brief shooting pain down one or both legs.
- A hollow piece of tubing, or epidural catheter, is inserted through the needle and secured in place with tape. Generally the tubing is very long and is taped up your back and over your shoulder.
- The anaesthetic is then injected through the tubing into the epidural space. Some women describe a sensation like cold water, while others

say it is like warm water running down your lower back and legs, as the medications take effect. The catheter means that top-ups of anaesthesia can be given if and when required.

- The whole thing takes only a few minutes and then, hopefully, any pain from your contractions will be gone!

EPIDURALS: FACT OR FICTION?

- 'You can't have an epidural until you are at least 4 centimetres.' Fiction: if you are in pain and feel you would like an epidural then ask your midwife for one. Guidance states that women should not be denied epidurals, even if they are in the latent stage of labour.

- 'If you wait too long, you won't be allowed an epidural.' Fiction: you can always ask for an epidural. Remember, though, that the drugs take up to 30 minutes to work, so if you are pushing and delivery is minutes away, you baby will arrive before it has time to work. However, there are other options for pain relief at this stage.

- 'Epidurals slow down labour.' Fiction: epidurals do not slow down the first stage of labour. Some studies have suggested that an epidural may slightly slow down the second stage but the epidurals in those studies may have involved higher doses of medication than is now generally used.

- 'If you have an epidural you won't know when to push.' Fiction: you may not feel any contractions with an epidural or you may feel some tightenings. Either way, you can still push the baby out as you or your midwife can feel when a contraction is occurring by putting a hand on your bump, which will go hard during a contraction, and you will be told to push.
- 'Epidurals mean you'll have to have forceps or a Caesarean.' Fiction: women with epidurals do have an increased chance of having an assisted delivery (forceps or ventouse), though this is performed only if necessary, for your or your baby's safety. Many women with epidurals push their babies out without any assistance. It may also be that women who request epidurals are having longer or more painful labours and are already at risk of needing a Caesarean. Again, remember many women have epidurals and deliver their babies naturally.
- 'The drugs used in epidurals affect the baby.' Fact: the medications used can affect the baby, making them slightly drowsy or, in the short term, can slow down the baby's breathing. However, epidurals are more effective and have fewer effects on the baby than pethidine injections. The medications used are safe in pregnancy.

- 'Epidurals always work, and leave you in no pain.'
  Fiction: although epidurals are very effective,
  there are no guarantees. Sometimes they produce
  a block that is patchy or more on one side of your
  body than the other, so you can still feel
  contractions on one side. This can often be
  corrected by changing your position. Very
  occasionally, an epidural will have to be resited.
  The medications used can also wear off, so you
  may need top-ups when the midwife injects more
  medication into the tube to bring relief. Each top-
  up can take up to 30 minutes to become effective.
- 'There is a risk of paralysis.' Mostly fiction: your
  legs may feel heavy and difficult to move when
  the epidural is in place, but with ambulatory
  epidurals this is less likely to happen. There is an
  extremely small risk of damage to nerves, which
  may leave you with a numb area on your legs or
  feet, or leg weakness; this occurs temporarily in
  about 1 in 1,000 epidurals. Permanent damage is
  even rarer, affecting only 1 in 13,000 epidurals.

The benefits of epidurals

After the long list of potential side-effects of epidurals (above), it is
perhaps worth mentioning again their potential benefits. They work.
In many cases you will be pain-free! Many women choose epidurals,
the main reason being that they are extremely effective at taking
away the pain of labour. If you are finding the pain difficult to cope
with, an epidural can transform your labour, making it bearable, even
painless or pleasurable!

'What a relief ... okay, so there was a bit of pushing and prodding to put the epidural in but in comparison to the pain of the contractions it was nothing! And then 20 minutes later, relief ... not totally pain-free as I still knew when contractions where coming but the pain went from being unbearable to being quite bearable. I could have a rest, and actually be involved in the labour instead of being consumed by the pain. I think the epidural calmed my husband down as well!' Mo, 26

Other regional blocks

- Spinal anaesthesia or spinal block – this is similar to an epidural block and is generally performed in theatre for Caesarean sections or other procedures.
- Pudendal block – involves injection of local anaesthetic into the skin of the vagina to block the transmission of pain (and touch) sensation in the lower half of the vagina. This is generally used for a forceps or ventouse delivery, or when an episiotomy (a cut made to help delivery) is needed, and the mother has not had an epidural (for more information on forceps and ventouse see page 285; on episiotomies see page 277). The local anaesthetic is temporary, generally lasting long enough for the baby to be delivered and for the midwife or doctor to stitch up any episiotomy or tears. It has no effect on the baby.

General anaesthesia

In rare circumstances, babies are delivered while the mother is under a general anaesthetic. This means that you will be unconscious while a Caesarean section is performed, just as you would be for any other operation. General anaesthetics can be used in certain obstetric emergencies, where time is of the essence to deliver the baby safely. An attempt may be made at a spinal block but if it is taking too long a general anaesthetic will be used.

Other circumstances include a maternal cause for performing the Caesarean under a general anaesthetic; for example, if the woman has a contraindication to a regional anaesthetic, such as certain blood-clotting problems. Finally, you may request a general anaesthetic if, for example, you have had a previous traumatic delivery or have an acute fear of childbirth. Please discuss this with your obstetric team.

Non-medical pain relief

Some of the following non-medical methods have more evidence of effectiveness than others. However, as long as you are not doing anything potentially harmful to the baby, you may find them helpful (check that your aromatherapy oils and so on are safe for pregnancy). Try to stay flexible – if you wanted a 'natural' delivery but have tried various options and feel that you want medication or an epidural then ask for them. Many women change their mind – after all, contractions are painful!

Breathing and relaxation techniques

The breathing and relaxation techniques described in earlier sections of this book can all be used during labour. Focusing on your breathing and using techniques to help you relax can ease the pain of labour, as pain is often worse when you are tense and scared. Using these techniques gives you something to focus on apart from the pain and can help keep you calm. Practise the techniques during your pregnancy so that they feel natural to you and you can perform them during your contractions. Perhaps one of the most important things to keep in mind during labour is the fact that every contraction brings you closer to the birth of your baby.

Water birth

A warm bath can be extremely relaxing and can help relieve pain during labour, especially in the early stages. Although water births may be less painful than those on dry land, there are risks such as the baby overheating (so the temperature of the water will be monitored), and it can also be more difficult to identify any problems. Therefore you may find that your unit will allow you to have a water birth only if there have been no problems in your pregnancy, and if you haven't taken any pethidine or have an epidural in place.

You can have a bath at home or in hospital. The water should be warm enough to be comfortable but not so hot that you have to lower yourself gingerly into the bath. You can use gas and air while in the water, and your baby will be monitored using a sonicaid or Pinard's stethoscope (see page 255). If you find the water helpful, most maternity units will consider offering you a water birth, where the baby is delivered in the water and quickly brought up to the surface. If you are considering a water birth you should inform your midwife in case any particular arrangements need to be made.

Massage

Massaging the lower back can relieve tension and help with the pain of contractions. Many people find that there is a type of healing or power that comes from being touched by another human; it is a physical reminder that you are not alone. It is also a method of involving your partner in the labour.

Transcutaneous electrical nerve stimulation (TENS)

A TENS machine delivers a small electric current through your skin. It is a small pack, generally battery powered, with pads that stick to your skin. The current feels like a tingling or pins-and-needles sensation, and you can control the strength of the frequency. The current blocks pain sensation and is also thought to stimulate the production of the body's feel-good hormones, endorphins, which act in the same way as painkillers by blocking the transmission of pain sensation to your brain.

TENS machines can be bought or hired from stores such as Boots for use during labour. They cannot be used in water so you can't use it in the bath or a birthing pool.

Acupuncture

Small needles are inserted into the skin at specific points. Acupuncture is a part of Chinese medicine, the philosophy of which is to do with balancing energy within the body. It is thought that acupuncture may also stimulate the production of endorphins to act as pain relief. You may have to find an appropriate acupuncturist yourself to treat you during your labour, though some hospitals do offer this service at certain hours.

Aromatherapy

The aromas of essential oils are used for various purposes. In labour, they can help you to relax. Oils can be used in a diluted form for massage, or can be inhaled using a vaporiser or in the bath. Be sure to check with an aromatherapist that the oils you intend to use are safe during pregnancy.

Reflexology

This involves massaging the feet and applying pressure to certain points. The philosophy behind reflexology is that the feet are a map of the rest of the body, and that by stimulating the feet, more distant parts of the body can be affected. You could ask a reflexologist to attend you in labour, or could teach some techniques to yourself or your partner.

Homeopathy

This uses extremely dilute active ingredients such as herbs, plants and minerals. Some women may find homeopathic remedies beneficial during labour. As they are so dilute many people consider them to be safe to use in pregnancy, though do check with your homeopathist.

Bach flower remedies

Here plants and flowers are taken as a tincture to relax you and dissipate stress. Check that the particular remedy you wish to use is safe for pregnancy and labour.

Hypnotherapy

Hypnosis can be performed by a hypnotherapist or you can, with practice, perform it on yourself. Using hypnotism, you will be encouraged to believe that the contractions are not painful.

> 'I really wanted to try for a natural birth, though I did know that I could change my mind if I needed to. So we hired the TENS machine, found out about water births and packed some massage oil in the hospital bag. Our birthing unit had an acupuncturist and he came in during the first stage of labour, which actually really helped me. By the time I was beginning to get tired and fed up I was 10 centimetres and my midwife said I could start pushing. I found that this totally rejuvenated me – now I could actually do something. More importantly, the end was in sight. Sure it hurt, really hurt, but I just kept saying to myself that each contraction would be the last and eventually it came true!' Amber, 27

THE SECOND STAGE

The second stage of labour is the pushing stage. It is generally considered to begin from the point when your cervix has dilated to 10 centimetres and you feel the urge to push and ends with delivery of the baby. It may also be called the stage of expulsion. As mentioned above, if you do feel the urge to push tell your midwife;

she will examine you to check that you are fully dilated before you can start pushing.

Up until now your contractions have caused your cervix to dilate and your baby to descend deep into your pelvis. These contractions will continue in the second stage, but now you will also need to work by pushing, adding to the force of the contractions forcing the baby down. The contractions are frequent – every two to three minutes for about one to one and a half minutes – so it can feel like there is little resting time in between.

During the second stage, your midwife will listen to the baby's heartbeat after every contraction. In some cases, such as if you have had an epidural, the baby's heart rate will be monitored continuously (for more information see page 255).

When and how to push

As the contraction reaches its peak you push and then rest until the next contraction occurs. If you have had an epidural you may not be aware of the contractions. In this situation your midwife will put her hand on your abdomen; when the contraction starts she will be able to feel your womb going very hard and will therefore be able to tell you when to push.

Pushing is not always quite as easy as it sounds, especially if you can't feel anything! Try to imagine that you are going to the toilet to open your bowels, or that you are bearing down, using your tummy muscles, helping to force the baby deeper into your pelvis and through the birth canal. You may find it easier if you brace your feet against the bed, your partner or midwife, so that you can push against something as you bear down.

Use your breath to help you, though don't hold your breath for the whole contraction as this may last quite a long time. Instead, you could try to count your breaths and therefore pushes, or ask your partner to count for you. For example, take a deep breath in and push for a count of five or ten, then breathe out. You may be able to fit in three or even four such breaths and therefore pushes with each contraction.

Think about pushing your baby down into your vagina with each push. Don't be embarrassed if you find that the pushing means you are grunting or shouting, or even passing a small amount of stool (which your midwife will simply and quietly remove; you may not even be aware of this). Your obstetric team has seen it all before.

The delivery

As the baby's head, or presenting part, is pushed through the pelvis the pain that you are experiencing may change. The contractions and their band of pressure around your abdomen will continue but you may also get a sensation of pressure in your bottom (as if you need to pass a stool). As the baby's head descends further, the skin of your vagina and perineum (area in between the vagina and anus) becomes very stretched. This can be painful, and is often described as a sharp stinging or burning sensation in and around your vagina. Delivering the baby will relieve this pain so think of every contraction as one contraction closer not only to delivering your baby but relief from any such pains.

At this point there is not long to go. The head will begin to appear with each contraction, though as the contractions and force from your pushing die away, the head slips back up the birth canal and away from view. As the contractions continue, combined with your pushing, the baby will descend further and the head stays visible between contractions. This is called crowning. You can put your hand down to feel the baby's head, or if you bring a mirror you can ask the midwife or your partner to show you the head. Your baby will be delivered shortly, probably in only a few more contractions.

It is important that the baby's head is delivered slowly, for the baby's safety and to decrease the risk of tearing, so try to listen to your midwife; if she asks you to stop pushing then try breathing in a short panting style and stop pushing until she tells you you can start again. Your midwife will be pressing against your perineum, generally with a piece of gauze, to try and prevent tears. There may be a longer gap than previously between contractions at this stage as there is less pressure on the cervix. Some women may even be advised that they need a drip of syntocinon (an artificial version of the natural hormone oxytocin) during this stage to stimulate contractions.

As the head is delivered your midwife will quickly check that the cord is not around the baby's neck; if it is she will lift it over the baby's head to prevent any problems. She may also wipe the baby's nose and mouth to remove any mucus or blood. The most common position for the baby to be in is face down, but once the head is free the baby will automatically stretch his neck and turn to face sideways. This means that the shoulders also face sideways so that they are narrower to fit more easily through the birth canal.

With the next contraction and your pushing, the baby's shoulders are delivered – first the uppermost shoulder and then the bottom one. The rest of the delivery is generally quick as the rest of the body slides out. The midwife will receive the baby and generally place him straight on to your tummy or into your arms, quickly drying him and covering him in a towel to keep warm. Your baby will look wet and be covered in amniotic fluid, blood and vernix. It is recommended that babies have direct skin-to-skin contact with you, where their skin touches yours. This helps control their body temperature, and encourages bonding and even breastfeeding. You can take as long as you like as long as everyone stays warm and snug!

'The pushing was quite difficult – when to push, how to push, how long to push ... I tried to listen to my midwife and ignore everything else, including the burning pain in my vagina. She said the only way to get rid of that was to push the baby out so I pushed and pushed and pushed!' Rebecca, 23

How long does the second stage last?

The second stage can last from a few minutes to a few hours, and on average lasts one hour. As with the first stage, the second stage is generally quicker in women who have previously delivered children. If the second stage lasts too long the woman's pushes will become less efficient as she gets tired, and there is a risk of damaging the pelvic floor from too much pushing. Long second stages are also associated with a risk of severe bleeding after delivery. Your obstetric unit will therefore have a policy regarding the second stage, and how long they allow women to push.

If you don't have an epidural you are generally allowed to push for about an hour. With an epidural, you will usually be allowed one hour of no pushing (where the baby passively descends into the birth canal) followed by one hour of pushing. After this point you will be assessed by your midwife or doctor and your options will be discussed. These may include continuing for a little longer or an assisted delivery, using forceps or a ventouse (for more information see page 285). If the foetus becomes stressed earlier in the second stage, as seen by a change in his heart rate, you will be seen by the medical team and assistance may be offered.

Tears and episiotomies

An episiotomy is a cut made in the vagina and perineum (skin between the vagina and anus). It is not carried out routinely during the second stage but may be recommended in certain cases, such as:

- if a forceps or ventouse delivery is needed
- if the skin of the perineum is very tight, more often in a first pregnancy
- for a breech baby
- for a very large baby

The skin is cleaned and then some local anaesthetic is injected (unless you have an epidural) before the incision is made. After

POSITIONS FOR THE SECOND STAGE

You may like to try different positions for the second stage to help with the contractions and for pushing. There is no 'correct' position, so you won't necessarily be lying down like you see in films; rather you will find the position that feels right for you.

- Sitting on the bed – sitting upright with your back supported by pillows. You might like to bend your legs, keep them open and hold on to your thighs as you push.
- Sitting on the bed – sitting upright or lying back slightly with your legs braced against the end of the bed or your partner and midwife as you push.
- Supported sitting – as described in the first stage, you sit in between your partner's legs, leaning back on to him for support.
- Squatting – you can squat on the floor with your back supported by the bed, or holding on to the bed or a chair. This position opens the hips and pelvis wide for delivery and allows gravity to help delivery.
- Semi-squatting – this has the same benefits as squatting but with more support. Your partner could sit on a chair or on the bed behind you and you sit on the floor on some pillows in between his knees. Your partner supports you by holding you under your arms.

- Kneeling – you could kneel on the bed, holding the upright back of the bed for support. Alternatively, you could kneel with your arms around your partner on one side and your midwife on the other to help support your weight. Or you may be comfortable supporting your own weight on your hands and knees. In this position you may find it comforting to rock slightly from side to side to help relieve some of the pressure symptoms.
- Supported standing – here you stand in front of your partner with your back to him; he supports you under your arms as you lean back on him and push down with your contractions.

delivery the episiotomy is repaired with dissolvable stitches; again you should not feel these as more local anaesthetic may be used. To perform the repair you will be asked to raise your legs in stirrups.

Episiotomies can be painful for a few days after delivery, so you will be given painkillers. Using icepacks can relieve some of the

'I had heard bad things about having an episiotomy and was really scared about tearing but actually I wasn't even aware that I had a tear until they told me I would need a few stitches. They then gave me some laxatives as I was a bit worried about going to the toilet, but apart from being a bit sore for a few days I was then completely back to normal.' Beth, 35

discomfort. Generally episiotomies do not cause any long-term problems and, for most women, the cut heals within a couple of weeks.

Tears can occur in the vaginal skin and perineum during delivery.
It is important to try and listen to your midwife and respond if she
asks you to stop pushing as this will be to try to reduce tearing as the
head is delivered. There are various degrees of tearing. Very minor
tears will heal on their own, though commonly stitches are required.
As with episiotomies, the body heals tears quickly, and in the vast
majority of cases there are no long-term problems.

FOR FATHERS (SECOND STAGE)

As the birth partner you continue to be important during the second
stage of labour, both physically and emotionally. Your partner may
find it helpful to lean on you, or for you to help prop her up in certain
positions. Alternatively she may like to push against you with her feet
during pushes. You may have already discussed where you would like
to be during the actual delivery, whether it is up by her head or holding her hand, or further down the bed where you can actually see the
baby being born.

Your partner may find verbal encouragement helpful, though be
warned that her mood might fluctuate. It is common for women who
five minutes ago were asking their partners for encouragement to
snap at them for doing what they were asked to do! She might like
you to help count her breaths and therefore her pushes, or just to
breathe with her to help keep her focused. She may get some relief
from a back massage, or just want you to hold her hand.

You might notice that your mother-to-be stops paying attention
to you or any other external factors during the second stage. It is
common for women to become very focused internally, almost going
into themselves as they focus on the task in hand. At this point they
may also become less self-conscious, perhaps as some instinctive,
even animal instinct about pushing and delivery takes over, and they
may grunt and heave as they push. This may be a way of dealing with

the pain, or it is simply instinctive; either way it probably means that delivery is very close.

> 'I might not have told him at the time but I was so glad he was there, not caring if I looked sweaty and had my face screwed up as I pushed, not expecting anything from me, just being there, supporting me, even if I did occasionally snap at him. And his face when he held the baby ...' Daisy, 23

THE THIRD STAGE

The third stage of labour begins after your baby is born and lasts until the delivery of the placenta and membranes. In general, as soon as the baby is born he is placed on your stomach or into your arms so that skin-to-skin contact can be made. At this stage the baby is still attached to you by his umbilical cord. The cord is cut by placing two clamps on it and cutting in between them; this prevents bleeding from either the baby or the placenta. Your midwife, your partner or even you could cut the cord between the two clamps. There will be a long length of cord attached to your baby; this is then shortened to a stump and a plastic clip is attached to it.

Management of the third stage will be one of the many aspects of labour your midwife will discuss with you when considering your birth plan. Traditional management does not involve the use of any medications, whereas active management does.

If no medications are used, there is often a gap of about 20–30 minutes after the baby is born until the placenta is delivered. During this stage contractions will continue and the placenta begins to separate from the wall of the womb, causing some bleeding. Once the placenta has separated, the contractions continue, squeezing the blood vessels to stop the bleeding. Signs that the placenta has separated include a gush of blood (the bleeding described above) and contractions. As these occur the umbilical cord will also look longer, as the placenta descends. Your midwife will be looking for these signs, and will then ask you to push at the same time as she pulls on the umbilical cord. She will have her other hand pushing on your lower abdomen, to keep your womb in place.

Once the placenta and membranes have been delivered, the midwife rubs your abdomen briskly and firmly. This rubbing stimulates or 'rubs up' more contractions, which then help to decrease bleeding as they squeeze the blood vessels. If your baby is already suckling at the breast during this stage (it is fine to do so, but also fine not to if you aren't ready or your baby isn't hungry), it also stimulates the body to produce the hormone oxytocin, which stimulates contractions.

Active management involves an injection of a medicine called syntometrine or syntocinon, generally into your thigh, as your baby's shoulders are delivered. Syntometrine contains syntocinon, the artificial version of the natural hormone oxytocin, to make your uterus contract, and ergometrine, which makes the contractions last a long time. The main reason for giving the injection is to reduce blood loss. This is important as the amount of bleeding can be significant and may even be dangerous. The separation of the placenta and membranes from the uterine wall is generally quicker in active management. The uterus stays contracted for a sustained period, up to about 45 minutes, reducing the amount of bleeding. As with traditional management, your midwife will gently pull on the cord while placing a hand on your lower abdomen.

The injection of syntometrine can lead to nausea or vomiting. Even if you have not had any medication it is common to become shaky after delivery, though this soon passes. The advantage of active management is that the third stage of labour is generally quicker and there is less risk of severe bleeding, though it is your choice. Put it in your birth plan or tell your midwife, though you will be asked for your permission before the injection is given.

Your midwife will then examine the placenta and membranes to check that they are intact and complete. Many women are so involved with their baby that they are not particularly aware of the goings-on of the third stage.

'I had completely forgotten that there was any more work to do! We were totally focused on our new baby girl. I remember I was marvelling at her tiny fingers when I had another contraction, was told to give another push and the placenta appeared.' Sally, 33

Potential complications in the third stage of labour

Complications can arise during the third stage of labour, including bleeding and problems delivering the placenta. If these problems do occur the medical team will be involved. They will discuss your care with you if action is required. Do bear in mind that, as with all parts of pregnancy and labour, in the majority of cases there are no problems and everything continues naturally.

Postpartum haemorrhage

A haemorrhage is when there is excessive bleeding. If you lose more than 500 millilitres of blood in the first 24 hours after delivery, this is called a primary postpartum haemorrhage. This is more common in traditional management of the third stage, and occurs in only about 5 per cent of women (1 in 20) who have active management of the third stage with the injection of syntometrine (see above).

Postpartum haemorrhage is most often due to the womb not contracting properly after the placenta has been delivered. It is more likely to happen in certain circumstances, such as after multiple deliveries, very long or very short deliveries or if you have had a postpartum haemorrhage in a previous pregnancy. The bleeding can also be due to tears in the vagina or other areas of the genitals (see page 277) or a retained placenta (see below).

If you do start bleeding, your midwife will ask other members of the obstetric team to come in and help assess and treat you. You may be given oxygen and a drip put in your arm to give you medication, fluids and, if necessary, blood. Depending on the amount of blood loss, various medications can be used to help stop the bleeding. Any tears to the vagina and surrounding tissues will be repaired. Rarely, if this isn't enough to stop the bleeding, you may be taken to theatre to have surgery to stop the bleeding, but most bleeding can be controlled.

A secondary postpartum haemorrhage is one that occurs between one day and six weeks after delivery. This is generally due to infection or a retained placenta and is treated depending on its cause, generally with antibiotics, or with a small surgical procedure to remove any retained placenta.

Retained placenta

This is when some or all of the placenta is left behind in the womb. It may cause bleeding or infection, which is why your midwife will check your placenta to see if it has all been delivered. If the placenta is retained after delivery medication may be used to try and help it come away, or it may need to be manually removed, generally in theatre. Often this is done by your doctor examining you vaginally and removing the placenta; occasionally surgery may be needed to remove all the placenta.

If you develop an infection or secondary postpartum haemorrhage in the weeks following delivery you may be offered an ultrasound scan. If fragments of the placenta or membranes (sometimes called products of conception) are seen you may be offered a surgical procedure called an ERPC (evacuation of retained products of conception) where these are removed under a general anaesthetic.

FOR FATHERS (THIRD STAGE)

You can continue to stay involved in the process of labour. You could, for example, cut the cord. Some men like to see the placenta after it has been delivered – the organ that sustained your baby in the womb. Of course, by this point you will probably want to hold both your partner and your baby!

ASSISTED DELIVERIES

An assisted delivery involves the use of forceps or vacuum extraction to help deliver the baby. If either of these is required you will still be involved in the labour – as you push with each contraction from above, the doctor will be assisting from below. In general, either forceps or ventouse deliveries are required if the second stage is very prolonged or if there are signs that the baby is becoming stressed or compromised. They can also be used for maternal reasons, such as the woman becoming exhausted from prolonged pushing, or due to maternal heart disease.

Each method has both advantages and disadvantages. Which will be the most appropriate will depend on your particular set of circumstances. In both cases you will be asked to lift your legs into what is called the lithotomy position – legs apart and in stirrups – to allow your doctors the best view of the birth canal and therefore access to your baby, though you can still sit up to help you push. Your bladder will be emptied quickly using a catheter. The catheter is then removed unless you have an epidural, in which case it may remain in place until you are able to be as mobile as normal.

Forceps

Generally an episiotomy will be needed. The blades (though these are not sharp) of the forceps are inserted one after the other into the vagina. They then lock together to form the forceps and cradle the baby's head. With every contraction you will push and your doctor will gently pull on the forceps to help guide the baby through the birth canal. The baby may be left with marks or bruises from the forceps on his face or head but these should fade. Babies' heads are often slightly misshapen or cone-like after delivery, and this may be more pronounced with forceps deliveries. This will resolve (see 'What will my baby look like?' page 296).

Vacuum extraction or ventouse

This involves using a vacuum to help guide the baby out. Here, an episiotomy is not always needed. A small plastic or metal cup is attached to the baby's head, and a vacuum created using a machine or hand-held pumping device attached to the cup. The vacuum ensures that the cup is firmly attached. With each contraction you will push while the doctor gently pulls on the handle or tubing of the cup to help guide the baby out. There is less risk of damage to the vaginal and perineal tissues with a ventouse than with a forceps delivery. In all cases, if your baby is born by ventouse, there will be a small swelling on his head where the cup was placed; this is called a chignon and resolves in a few days. In approximately one in 20 cases the baby develops bleeding just beneath the skull from the effect of the cup. This is generally mild and tends to resolve spontaneously in a couple of weeks without any long-term problems.

Your doctor will decide whether a forceps or ventouse delivery is appropriate for you, depending on the presentation of the baby and how well descended he is. Some doctors feel that a ventouse is less likely to be successful if this is your first pregnancy. In some circumstances a doctor may attempt a ventouse delivery, but if this is not successful will change to use forceps to deliver the baby.

Commonly, if you have an assisted delivery a paediatrician will be present in the room at the time of delivery. The baby is generally placed on your tummy while the cord is cut, and then the baby is quickly handed to the paediatrician to be checked. As long as there are no problems you will soon be given your baby to hold.

Remember, although there may suddenly be lots of people in your delivery room and lots of equipment being opened and used, assisted deliveries are performed regularly if it is decided that it is the safest method of delivering your baby. There is a misconception that they are a bad thing, that you have given in to a doctor. However, that is not the case. A decision is made with you about the safety of you and your baby. Don't let anyone make you feel guilty that you did not give birth without any assistance. Indeed, you are a good parent who made an appropriate decision about the health of your child.

> 'Having forceps wasn't really part of my birth plan but when they told me that the baby's heart rate was going down I would have done anything if it meant that she would be safe. I didn't feel it as I had an epidural, and a few pushes later it was all done. To be honest, it was the number of people in the room that scared me more than anything else but after a quick check over they gave her back to me and all left! Then it was just us ...' Tara, 32

CAESAREAN SECTIONS

Caesarean section rates vary, but approximately 20 per cent or one in five babies are born by Caesarean. This rate has been increasing, and possible reasons for this include:

- Better foetal monitoring during labour so that compromised babies are identified more effectively
- Increasing number of multiple pregnancies

- Women with certain pre-existing medical conditions having babies

The main reason for the increase in the number of Caesareans is probably the rise in the number of women choosing to have a Caesarean after having a section in a previous pregnancy.

Elective Caesarean

An elective Caesarean is one that is planned in advance, if it is thought that a Caesarean is safer than a vaginal delivery. Reasons include:

- a multiple pregnancy
- a breech baby
- a low-lying placenta (placenta praevia, see page 206)
- severe pre-eclampsia (see page 155)
- another medical condition that would make vaginal delivery risky

If you have had a previous Caesarean section you may choose to have an elective one for any subsequent pregnancies, though many women have natural births after a Caesarean – this is called a vaginal birth after Caesarean (VBAC), and used to be called a trial of scar. Your antenatal team will discuss your options with you.

If you are having an elective Caesarean you will be asked not to eat or drink anything from midnight the previous night and come into hospital, probably early in the morning. You will also be given a medication called ranitidine to take, to stop your stomach producing acid. This, combined with your stomach being empty, is thought to be safer in case a general anaesthetic is needed (though this is rare).

Emergency Caesarean

An emergency Caesarean, conversely, is one that has not been planned in advance but is decided on at the time if, for example, the baby is becoming compromised. As with any procedure, if your midwife and medical team feel that a Caesarean is the safest option to deliver your baby, this will be discussed with you.

There are degrees of 'emergency' Caesarean section. These range from the section which is decided on due to a failure of labour to progress but the baby is not compromised to the rarer situation where the delivery needs to occur rapidly to ensure the safety of the baby and mother.

What happens in a Caesarean?

A Caesarean section is a major operation with a significant recovery time. The risks of a Caesarean include bleeding, infection and the development of blood clots (you will be given a small injection daily after the operation to try and prevent these). These risks have to be weighed up against the safe delivery of the baby.

The Caesarean will be carried out in an operating theatre. You will be asked to remove your jewellery and, if you are not already in one, put on a gown. Your partner can be with you during the Caesarean; he will be asked to change his clothes and will be loaned a pair of sterile scrubs (trousers and a top), shoes and a disposable hat. An anaesthetist will come to assess you and will insert a drip into your arm to give you fluids. If you are having an emergency section you may already have an epidural; if so, this will be topped up to ensure that you are pain free. If you don't already have pain relief, for example if you are having an elective section, the anaesthetist will insert a spinal or epidural (for more information see page 263). The anaesthetist will check that the anaesthetic is working by spraying you with a cold spray; when you cannot feel the spray as cold it is safe for the procedure to begin.

A urinary catheter is always inserted if you have a Caesarean to keep your bladder empty. Your epidural or spinal anaesthetic will affect your ability to be mobile and walk to the toilet; the catheter means that you don't have to get up and go to the toilet for the first 24 hours or so after the operation, and won't be removed until you are mobile again. Your skin is then cleaned and sterile drapes put over your legs and upper abdomen. A screen is made using these drapes so you and your partner (who can sit by your head) cannot see the procedure.

The incision made during a Caesarean is just below your bikini line, where your pubic hair begins, so that the hair may hide some of the scar. The surgeon then delivers the baby and the screen is lowered so that you can see your baby. As he is delivered you may feel some pushing or odd sensations in your tummy, which are generally not painful. The screen is then raised, the cord clamped and cut and the baby handed to a midwife or paediatrician to be checked over. The baby is then wrapped and handed to you or your partner. While that is happening the surgeon will be closing the incision with stitches, though you will probably be too wrapped up in your baby to pay much attention!

The length of time a Caesarean takes will depend on the anaesthetist, surgeon and reason for the procedure. The majority of the time is spent inserting and waiting for the anaesthetic to take effect, and suturing you up again after the delivery. Delivering the baby does not take long at all! You will then be transferred through to recovery, where a midwife will observe you closely for a few hours before you are transferred to the postnatal ward.

'I had to have a Caesarean as I started bleeding and they were worried about the baby. It was quite a strange experience, as I couldn't really feel anything apart from some pushing and prodding around. Instead of the long labour I had been gearing myself up for, about 30 minutes later they handed me my baby!' Christina, 35

MULTIPLE BIRTHS

The rate of multiple (twin, triplet or even more!) pregnancies has risen over recent years, mainly due to fertility treatments. If you are carrying a multiple pregnancy you will be closely monitored as you are more likely to develop complications such as premature labour or growth restriction, where one or more of the babies is small for its age.

Twins are the commonest type of multiple pregnancy and can be delivered vaginally, though close monitoring is required. For the babies to be delivered vaginally, the first baby should be head down. If the lowest baby is lying sideways (transverse) it will not be possible to have a vaginal delivery as the baby won't have room to turn. The position of the second baby, be it head up or down or sideways, can change after the first baby is born. Each unit may have a slightly different policy but, in general, delivery of the second twin should be within 30 minutes of delivery of the first; if this does not look possible you may be advised to have an emergency Caesarean.

Rather than delivering the babies vaginally, you will be offered the choice of an elective Caesarean section. You may be advised to book an elective Caesarean if, for example, the babies are growth restricted or the first twin is breech. A paediatrician will be present at the delivery, be it vaginal or Caesarean, and the babies checked over immediately.

BREECH DELIVERIES

Although as many as one in four babies will be in a breech position at an earlier stage of pregnancy (see Week 28), only approximately 4 per cent of babies are breech at term. There are various breech positions depending on whether the buttocks or the feet are the presenting (lowest) part.

Breech deliveries are considered to be more risky than cephalic (head-down) deliveries as there are various risks, such as the cord falling through the cervix, and a slow labour as the soft buttocks don't stimulate the cervix in the same way as the baby's head. You will be offered external cephalic version at around 37 weeks in an attempt to turn the baby (see page 217). If this doesn't work you may be advised that a Caesarean is the safest form of delivering your baby, depending on your particular set of circumstances. If that is not the case and you go into labour, both you and your baby will be closely monitored throughout.

An episiotomy is commonly performed. At the time of delivery your midwife or doctor will help deliver the baby, generally its buttocks first, then legs, followed by the trunk and shoulders and then the head. Forceps may be applied to help guide the head out safely. If at any point the baby's heart rate patterns become suspicious you may be advised to have a Caesarean section.

PREMATURE LABOUR

Premature labour is one that occurs earlier than 37 weeks' gestation. For more information, see Week 32.

the hours immediately after birth

You will be given plenty of time to hold and cuddle your baby, to have skin-to-skin contact with him and allow him to feed. He will be dried and wrapped to help him keep warm, but there are also some first checks to be carried out.

APGAR SCORES AND EXAMINATION

After the baby is delivered and placed on your tummy or in your arms, your midwife will quickly assess his condition, at one minute and at five minutes after delivery. This assessment uses the Apgar score, which looks at heart rate, skin colour, breathing, muscle tone and reflexes. The maximum score is ten – two points in each area. A score over seven generally means that the baby is in good condition, and does not need medical help, for example with breathing; a lower score indicates that help is needed. The score does not predict any long-term effects in your baby, just whether immediate action is needed.

After your first cuddles, your midwife will probably weigh the baby and measure his length and head circumference (widest point around the head), though this does not have to be done at this point and can wait until the first baby check by the paediatrician before you leave hospital. The midwife will also check the baby, including listening to the heart and lungs, checking the spine and counting fingers and toes. A further check will be carried out by a paediatrician before you leave hospital, and your GP will repeat the examination eight weeks after delivery.

IDENTIFICATION

Plastic identification tags will be attached to your baby's ankles and wrists. The information written on the tags includes your surname, your hospital number and your baby's hospital number. You will be given a tag that also has your and your baby's hospital numbers on it. This is so that your baby can be clearly identified as yours! The cot may also be labelled with your baby's surname and both your hospital numbers. Don't worry if you haven't got a first name for your baby yet; he will be identified as 'Baby', followed by your surname.

VITAMIN K

Vitamin K is an essential component in the body which clots our blood, preventing bleeding. It is generally obtained through the diet, but babies do not get much vitamin K from milk. The liver is involved in the mechanism of clotting your blood, and in babies is immature so it may not work very efficiently. These two factors mean that babies have a risk of internal bleeding, called haemorrhagic disease of the newborn (or vitamin K deficiency bleeding). Therefore, it is recommended that all babies receive supplements of vitamin K after birth.

Vitamin K can be given by injection soon after birth (into the baby's thigh), or orally, though if oral doses are given they need to be repeated – two doses in the first week followed by one last dose at one month. Most babies are given the injection so only one dose is needed.

'The first hour or so after the birth are a bit of a blur really. I remember that the midwife checked the baby. He was weighed and things and then we made some phone calls to people, but really all I remember is holding him; holding him and actually saying hello for the first time.' Freya, 27

YOUR (ALREADY!) CHANGING BABY

Even as your baby is taking his first breath, various changes are happening in his body to adapt him to life where he has to breathe for himself and does not receive a supply of oxygen from you via the umbilical cord. That first breath or gasp can take place as early as when only the head has been delivered and the rest of his body is still within the birth canal. This is triggered by the change in environment – the outside world is colder and much lighter than the womb. The cutting of the cord, stopping the supply of oxygen from you, also stimulates breathing.

In the womb, your baby did not need to send all his blood to his lungs to receive oxygen as he was getting it from you. Now, even with his first breath, changes are made in his heart and circulatory system so that blood is sent to the lungs to receive oxygen before returning to the heart to be pumped to the rest of the body.

Not only is your baby no longer receiving his oxygen supply from you, but he no longer receives glucose either. While waiting for your milk supply to become well established, he uses the stores of a substance called glycogen that has been built up in his liver during pregnancy, turning it into glucose for energy.

Finally, now he is in the outside world he has to learn to control his own temperature. You will help him by ensuring he is wrapped up warmly. He has also laid down a supply of a special kind of fat in the womb, called brown fat, which he can now use to supply him with heat.

And all these changes occur without either you or your baby knowing anything about it!

'WHAT WILL MY BABY LOOK LIKE?'

The image of the newborn baby, all soft skinned and sweet smelling, generally does not occur straight after delivery! No matter how the baby is delivered he will emerge covered in amniotic fluid, some vernix and often some of your blood. The fluids are dried off but the vernix is generally not removed as it is protective for the skin; it may take a few days to fully disappear, though it can be rubbed into the baby's skin. There may still be some lanugo hair present, often on the shoulders and upper arms (especially if the baby is premature), which will also disappear with time. Babies are generally born with blue eyes, as the pigment has not been fully deposited to darken them; the colour of baby's eyes can change for many months after birth.

If you had a natural delivery, the baby's head may be elongated due to the bones overlapping to allow the head to be compressed slightly as it passed through the birth canal. If you had a forceps delivery, there may be marks from the forceps on the head or face, and the elongation of the head may also be pronounced. After a ventouse delivery there may be a swelling on the baby's head. These marks will all fade over a few days. If you run your hands gently over

'I didn't care that he came out covered in gunk and that his head was a bit of a funny shape. They dried him off and he was mine, my baby, perfect to me.'
Michelle, 30

your baby's head you will notice that there appears to be a small gap, or softer part, at the back and top of his head. These are called the fontanelles and are the spaces that allowed his bones to overlap as he passed through the birth canal. There is a tough fibrous covering protecting your baby's brain so normal handling of your baby shouldn't cause any problems. However, avoid applying direct pressure on to the fontanelles. These fontanelles gradually shrink and close over many months.

the postpartum period

The postnatal or postpartum period starts after labour has finished and the baby has been delivered and lasts for the six weeks after the baby is born. It is a time of great change – not just the physical changes occurring in your body, but emotional changes too, as you and all the people close to you adjust to having a new baby.

GOING HOME AND POSTNATAL CHECKS

How long you will be advised to stay in hospital depends on the method of delivery and whether or not there are any complications. If this is your first baby you may stay in hospital for slightly longer so that the midwives can support you and show you how to breastfeed and give your baby a bath. On average, women who have had a vaginal birth tend to spend a night in hospital after delivery but the stay can be as short as six hours! If you have had a Caesarean you will be advised to stay in hospital for at least three days as the recovery period is slower. You will also be advised that you cannot drive for six weeks after the operation and should avoid lifting anything heavier than your new baby as you recover.

While in the hospital your baby will be checked over by a paediatrician. The doctor will examine your baby from head to toe, looking at every organ system: the colour of his skin, activity, breathing pattern, head, eyes, mouth, heart, fingers and toes, lungs, tummy, genitals, hips and reflexes.

Visits by your community midwife

When you go home you will be visited by a community midwife. She will visit as often as needed, ideally daily, for the first week to 10 days or so after delivery (though sometimes visits are only every two or three days). She will support you at home, help you with breastfeeding and answer any questions you may have. She will also weigh the baby (she will bring a set of scales to your house) on approximately Day 5 and then again on approximately Day 10. Babies tend to lose weight in the first few days after birth while waiting for your milk supply to be established; they are designed to cope with this and use their stores of fat for energy. If, however, the baby has lost more than 10 per cent of his birth weight at Day 5, you will be advised to see a doctor. Your baby will then be weighed again on approximately Day 10 to check that he is gaining weight.

Your midwife will also carry out a 'heel-prick' or Guthrie test within the first two weeks of birth, again generally on approximately Day 5 or 6, once the baby is feeding well and the milk supply is established. This test involves pricking the baby's heel with a very tiny needle; many mothers choose to feed their babies while the test is being performed and the babies barely appear to notice the prick. Drops of blood are placed on a special card and are screened for rare but important diseases. These conditions include:

- hypothyroidism – a deficiency of thyroid hormone causing growth problems and learning difficulties
- phenylketonuria – a condition where the body cannot digest a certain amino acid in protein
- sickle cell anaemia – which affects red blood cells

- cystic fibrosis – which mainly affects the lungs and digestive tract
- medium-chain-acyl-CoA dehydrogenase deficiency (MCADD) – a rare disease where the body cannot turn fat into energy

Some of these conditions are easily treatable with diet or medication; others are not but medical intervention will still be needed. The Newborn Screening Programme aims to pick up cases early and treat where possible. The screening committee is considering extending the screening programme to include other conditions.

Your midwife will hand over the care of you and your baby to your local health visitor once you both feel that you are coping well at home. Your health visitor will initially come to see you at home and is there to support you. You will be given the contact numbers of your health visitor and can phone them to ask questions. In general, after the initial assessment, you can then see your health visitor either by appointment or at your local baby clinic. Remember that if you have any concerns you can also make an appointment to see your GP.

YOUR CHANGING BODY

Throughout pregnancy your body was changing and adapting to compensate for your developing baby. Your abdominal organs shifted and even your lungs were squashed to accommodate the growing uterus. Your womb increased in size dramatically and your breasts changed. Your blood volume increased and all your blood vessels dilated to prevent you developing high blood pressure. The hormones of pregnancy affected every part of your body from your skin to your hair, and may have affected your mood. These changes took nine months, or the length of your pregnancy. After the baby is born, your changing hormone levels make everything change back within approximately six weeks!

The amount of blood in your circulatory system will decrease to its pre-pregnancy volume, and with it your blood vessels also narrow back to their normal size so that your blood pressure doesn't fall. This extra volume and any extra fluid in your body will be absorbed and then urinated out.

'I've gone through labour. Why am I still getting tummy pains?'

Your uterus will slowly shrink down, though it may remain slightly bigger than previously. Initially, as your womb shrinks you may get some cramping pains, sometimes called after pains, which generally only occur in the first few days after birth. You may notice them when you are breastfeeding because the hormone oxytocin is released, which also makes your uterus contract. You can take painkillers such as paracetamol to help with any pain.

'I'm bleeding. Is this my period already?'

You will be bleeding, like a period, after delivery. This discharge is called lochia and is the lining of your womb being shed. This bleeding lasts longer than a period, perhaps for up to a few weeks, though it gradually gets lighter and lighter. You can buy maternity pads or sanitary towels. Using pads means that you can monitor how much you are bleeding; you should not use tampons after you give birth until your next period because infection is more likely with tampons. If you are still bleeding after your six-week check, or if the bleeding gets heavier instead of lighter or becomes very offensive in smell and you have pains in your lower abdomen, contact your GP as you may have developed an infection.

Your breasts

Your breasts will also change. As soon as your placenta has been delivered, your breasts will start to produce colostrum. Your milk comes in on around Day 3 or 4 after delivery; at this point many women find that their breasts become swollen and engorged and can feel very tender (for more information about breastfeeding see page 310).

Pelvic floor muscles

Both pregnancy and childbirth weaken the pelvic floor muscles, so you may notice that you leak small amounts of urine, especially if you cough or sneeze, though doing your pelvic floor exercises regularly from now on should help prevent this occurring (for more information see page 91). Try and do them at least once daily, such as whenever you brush your teeth, or you could do them during breastfeeding.

Body shape

Your body shape will also change. Immediately after the birth your bump will have shrunk, though you won't be back to your pre-pregnancy shape straight away. Your body may not return to exactly the same shape and condition as previously; you may, for example, have stretch marks. With time, a healthy diet and plenty of exercise you should be able to lose the weight gained in pregnancy; breastfeeding uses extra calories, which can help with weight loss. It is

'I felt like if I saw one more picture of a celebrity mum who lost all her baby weight in three weeks after her delivery I would start screaming! It is so unrealistic. Three weeks after Jake was born I was proud if I found the time to have a shower, never mind go to the gym. And I was hungry, really hungry. Breastfeeding made me starving. I tried not to eat junk and then just ignored the pictures of skinny women in the press. It took months, actually months and months, for the weight to go. The impression these celebs give is wrong. Most people don't lose their weight that fast and you shouldn't feel bad about it!' Casey, 27

important not to rush: it takes different women different amounts of time to lose the weight, and there is a lot of pressure from the media for the change to be almost instantaneous.

EMOTIONAL CHANGES

Just as your body is going through lots of changes, you are also experiencing lots of mental and emotional upheaval. Firstly, you have gone through labour, which leaves most women drained and tired, both physically and mentally. Then, your changing hormone levels can affect how you feel. Combined with this, you are dealing with the demands of a newborn baby and lack of sleep!

Although you have spent nine months preparing for the birth of your baby, the reality of a newborn can be overwhelming. It is common for women to feel scared or powerless. Many are anxious about whether they are doing the right thing, or that they don't match up to the picture they had spent so long imagining during their pregnancy. Try to remember that you are doing your best and

BONDING

You are developing a new relationship with your baby. Many women feel they should instantly 'bond' with their baby, that there should be an instantaneous rush or hit of love. For some women this is the case, but for many the process is a slow and gradual one as it takes time for the two of you to get to know each other.

will be the best mother for your baby, and that these feelings are extremely common.

Having a baby will affect all your relationships, from that with your partner to those with your friends. Some people may find it difficult to understand that your focus will be on your baby and how busy you can be with a newborn. Your partner may also find this difficult and might be feeling tired and strained from being woken in the night by the baby but still having to go to work in the daytime. Keep talking to each other! Partners can also feel left out, so try to encourage him to spend as much time as possible with the baby, changing nappies or giving cuddles (for more information see 'For Fathers', page 317).

> 'I remember holding him and waiting for the rush that everyone talks about, the one where you look into their eyes and instantly love them. And I waited, and then I cried because I thought that as I didn't feel it I must be a bad mother. I wanted to look after him and protect him but although he'd been in me for nine months I didn't know him. How can you love something you don't know? He is now 11 months old and I am constantly astounded at how happy he makes me and how much I love him, but it wasn't instant.' Rowena, 32

Baby blues

Many women feel very weepy in the first week or so after delivery. This is known as the 'baby blues'. It tends to coincide with the time that the milk comes in, around Day 3–5, and can last a couple of weeks. The baby blues are probably due to a combination of factors:

- changing hormone levels
- physical discomfort from your after pains or stitches; your breasts may also be sore and engorged
- tiredness after labour and a lack of sleep at night

You may find that your emotions swing quite rapidly, that you can be happy and laughing one minute and crying the next. These surges of emotion can make you feel overwhelmed, or you may be guilty that you are feeling down when you should be joyful that you have a baby. Rest assured that this tends to settle down within a few weeks as your body adjusts both mentally and physically to the changes after delivery. Talk to your partner, mother or friends. Cry if and when you need to, and try and remember that things will generally get better soon.

'The baby blues took us both by surprise. Okay, she had got pretty emotional during the pregnancy, crying at things on the telly, but three days after the baby was born she wailed all day, literally all day, and I got really worried. Next day, back to normal – bizarre!' Sean, 31

Siblings

Siblings commonly find the arrival of a new brother or sister difficult, so try to include them as much as possible. Many siblings may respond by becoming more attention-seeking, naughty or clingy. This is a normal reaction. Young children find it difficult to express their emotions (as can adults), and their confusion and anxieties regarding such a big change in their lives can show as changes in their behaviour. This stage will hopefully pass as they get used to the new baby.

You can help to prepare siblings for the arrival of their brother or sister by talking about the baby in your bump and explaining to them what is going to happen. Even if they don't seem to understand or even be listening to you very much, with lots of repetition they will begin to understand.

Involve them as much as possible, perhaps asking if they would like to choose a present for the baby, or which colour babygro they think the baby will like. Giving siblings a new role as the special older sister or brother with a new job to do can help them feel involved, even if it is something as simple as making sure that their teddies are lined up neatly ready for the baby to see, or making a card for the baby.

When you do bring your baby home, try to keep the older sibling interested as much as possible. How much they can do will depend on their age, but perhaps they can hand you the nappy cream or a nappy during changing, or read a story to you while you are feeding. Make sure that you also spend some one-to-one time with your older child or children so that they continue to feel special and loved.

Postnatal depression

Postnatal depression is different from the baby blues in that it does not get better in a few weeks after delivery. It can occur at any point during the first year and can range from very mild to severe depression. It is not known what causes postnatal depression, though if you have had an episode of postnatal depression in the past you are more likely to develop it again.

Symptoms of depression include:

- feeling persistently low or down
- feeling that things are hopeless
- feeling weepy or crying regularly
- feeling worthless or a failure to yourself or your family
- tiredness
- difficulty sleeping, such as waking up very early in the morning and not being able to get back to sleep
- loss of appetite
- loss of libido (sex drive)
- difficulty concentrating

Postnatal depression is an illness and is not your or anyone's fault. It can be difficult to recognise these symptoms in yourself but if you do feel that you are depressed, or your partner or family feels so, speak to your doctor or midwife who will be looking for these signs at every check. The treatment for postnatal depression depends on the severity of the illness and includes giving increased support, counselling and antidepressants (medication can be given which is safe for breastfeeding).

Even if you do not develop depression, it is common for new mothers to have periods of feeling exhausted and unable to cope. Try to surround yourself with supportive family and friends, such as other women you may have met during antenatal classes who really understand what you are going through. You could try to meet new mothers by attending local mother and baby groups; this also helps you to get out of the house. Ask your friends or health visitor or contact your council's children's information service for details of local groups.

Try to sleep when you can. When the baby sleeps in the day you should also try to rest. Doing some gentle exercise and eating healthily can also help you to feel good. You are not alone – ask for help when you need it, and don't feel guilty about doing so. Your health visitor and GP can be very helpful so do contact them, though they will also be asking you questions about your mood at your checkups.

'My friends really didn't get it. They wanted me to go out with them, as if she wasn't here, but I couldn't – apart from the fact that I was breastfeeding I was too exhausted. I started going to local mothers' groups instead and found that they really 'got' me. It was a big relief to be able to talk to people that understood and didn't make me feel guilty.' Meg, 22

Your GP can refer you to a counsellor or a psychologist, who can also help you deal with your emotions. Help can be anything from talking to a friend, your mum walking the baby for an hour so you can rest, to seeing your doctor and asking for therapy or medication.

Puerperal psychosis

This condition is rare, occurring in about one to two women out of a thousand. Here women can be confused or agitated and may have delusions or hallucinations. This tends to start in the first two weeks after delivery and is a serious condition. If you feel that you or your partner is affected then contact your doctor as soon as possible. The condition is treated with medication.

YOUR CHANGING BABY

Babies change, develop and grow very rapidly within the first few years of life. You will even begin to notice some changes within the first six weeks or so. If you do have any concerns then speak to your health visitor or GP.

Your baby's head will probably change shape slightly, especially if it was elongated due to the effects of delivery. Any other signs from the delivery, such as marks on the face, should fade. He will probably lose weight in the first few days of life while waiting for the milk supply to be established but will then begin to put on weight steadily – you may even have to go up quickly to the next size of babygro or nappy!

After delivery the umbilical stump will be clamped to a short length with a plastic clamp; this should be left on. Within a few days the cord will begin to shrivel, blacken and dry out, and falls off generally in the first few weeks after birth. The stump should be kept clean and dry. Some newborn nappies are designed so that the stump is left free; if not, fold over the top of the nappy so the stump isn't enclosed and doesn't get urine or stool on it. If it does get dirty you can clean it with water.

When the stump falls off you may notice a very small amount of bleeding in the nappy, which is normal. The site will heal over after the stump falls off in about a week. If your baby develops a fever, the stump becomes very smelly or the skin around the belly button becomes red and inflamed, he may have developed an infection in the stump so see your doctor. In about one in 50 cases a red lump will form underneath; this is called an umbilical granuloma and generally heals on its own but do see your doctor if you are worried. In the majority of cases the stump dries up, shrivels and falls off on its own without problems.

You will also notice that your baby's poo changes over the first few weeks of life. Initially the stool looks dark brown/green in colour and is very thick and sticky. This is the meconium and is made up of swallowed amniotic fluid, bile and other cells. As your milk supply is established, the stool will change, often becoming a bright mustard yellow in colour and very liquid – it may even look like it has little mustard seeds in it! Formula-fed babies can have varying colours of stool.

Babies can produce surprising amounts of poo so don't worry if you are changing five or six dirty nappies a day. The colour itself can also vary from that described above. If, however, there is blood in the stool or it is black or completely white, see your doctor.

Even though your baby is still so young you may notice that he can hear and see. Initially your baby may startle to a loud noise, and within a few weeks will begin to quieten to your voice or to a prolonged noise like the vacuum cleaner. Babies are born very short-sighted but can see well enough to see your face while you feed them. Within a few weeks you will notice that your baby fixes on your face and will follow it if you move slightly. Many babies have a squint during the first few weeks of life, but if they are still squinting at your postnatal check, mention it to your doctor. Perhaps one of the biggest milestones in the first few weeks of life is the first responsive smile. This generally occurs at approximately six weeks and makes it all worthwhile!

BREASTFEEDING

Breastfeeding has many benefits, ranging from decreasing the risk of allergies to passing on antibodies to protect the baby from infection, and helping the development of the nervous system. It also helps you to lose your baby weight and helps protect you from certain cancers, such as ovarian cancer and breast cancer. It contains all the nutrients your baby needs and can help with the bonding process. It is also cheap, portable and easily accessible!

For the first few days after delivery your breasts will produce a substance called colostrum. This is high in protein and antibodies to help protect your baby from infection. The milk then 'comes in' at around Day 3 or 4, and you may notice your breasts feel very full and heavy. Initially, it is a combination of milk and colostrum, and within a few weeks it will just be milk.

Breastfeeding is a natural process but it is not always as easy as it looks, at least initially! It may take some time and practice for both you and your baby to learn how to breastfeed. Ask your midwife or a breastfeeding counsellor to show you how best to position the baby. Breastfeeding should not be a painful process, though it is common for there to be some discomfort as the baby attaches for the first few feeds; this should quickly pass and if it does not then ask for help as the baby may not be latching on properly. You may wish to purchase some breast or nipple pads and nipple cream. Breast pads are small pads that you insert into your bra. They absorb any leakages, keeping your breasts dry. Nipple cream can be soothing if you have sore nipples.

For successful breastfeeding, start with 'tummy to tummy' – turn the baby so he is lying on his side with his tummy facing yours. Then tickle the baby's upper lip or nose with your nipple and wait until he opens his mouth really wide before moving him on to the breast. He should be taking in the nipple and lots of the areola; his bottom lip should be curled outwards and you should be able to see more areola above his top lip than below his bottom lip – this means that the nipple will be pointing upwards in his mouth.

Signs of successful feeding are that there is no discomfort; the baby initially sucks rapidly but then changes to long sucks and you can both see and hear the baby swallowing. You may also notice the 'let-down' reflex – after your baby has been sucking for a few seconds the milk comes down into the ducts and out through the nipple and you get a tingling or warm sensation in your breasts. Let your baby feed as long as he wants to, and feed him when he asks for it by crying!

Expressing milk

You may wish to try expressing breast milk. This can be stored in the fridge or freezer in breast milk freezer bags or in bottles. Some women like to express milk so that their partner can give a feed, such as at night or so that they can go out or simply have a rest. Expressing can take a little practice, so don't be surprised if you only get a little milk at first. Remember, too, that your breasts will only be producing as much as your baby is drinking, so you will get less milk when your baby is a newborn than when he is six months old!

You can express by hand, gently massing each breast then rolling or squeezing your nipple between your thumb and finger. Many women find it both easier and quicker to use a breast pump, which can be manual or electric. These pumps try to simulate the action of the baby suckling to stimulate the let-down reflex. Expressed milk kept at room temperature (no hotter than 25°C) can be kept for up to

'For me, breastfeeding was the obvious answer. It is so convenient, portable, instantly ready and warm, and cheap! Apart from that, though, it was my time with her, time where I couldn't do anything else apart from look at her, and look at her looking at me, and I loved it.' Ruth, 29

four hours; in a fridge (4°C or colder) up to three days and in a freezer up to three months.

BOTTLE FEEDING

While breast milk is considered the best way to feed your baby, there are various reasons why you might choose to use bottles instead. Your doctor may have advised you to bottle feed if, for example, you have HIV or if the baby has specific difficulties with sucking and feeding. If you are not producing enough breast milk your doctor may have advised you to top the baby up with formula milk. Perhaps the most common reason, however, is that breastfeeding may not fit in with your lifestyle. Bottle feeding allows you more freedom if, for example, you are returning to work, or if your partner would like to share the feeding (though you could express some breast milk into a bottle).

Bottle feeding means that anyone can feed the baby and you know exactly how much he is getting. However, it is more expensive, and time and care has to be taken to sterilise the bottles, make up formula and heat the milk correctly. Babies who are bottle fed can still be fed on demand. If, though, you are thinking about giving up breastfeeding because you are finding it uncomfortable, or you think you aren't doing it right, then ask for help from your midwife, a breastfeeding counsellor or health visitor.

You will need to purchase a steriliser or sterilising tablets so you can sterilise all the bottles and teats after each use to prevent infection. Wash the bottles first with hot water and detergent to remove any milk, then rinse well. Many women choose to wash their bottles after each use and then sterilise them all in one batch, so all the bottles are clean for the next day.

You can purchase baby formula from most supermarkets and pharmacies, in both ready-prepared and powder forms. The formulas are made to try to match breast milk as closely as possible. The ready-prepared versions are more expensive but the milk is ready to use; the

UNIVERSAL NEWBORN HEARING SCREEN

You will be offered a hearing test for your baby. One or two babies in a thousand have hearing loss, which affects their development of language and social skills. It is important to pick it up early so that appropriate help and support can be given. In some units, you will be offered the hearing test while you are in hospital; in others, the test is carried out in the community within a few weeks or so of birth.

The official name of the test is otoacoustic emission testing. It is not uncomfortable and involves placing a small earpiece into the baby's ear while they are asleep or feeding (and therefore quiet). A sound is sent into the ear, which is reflected back by the eardrum in a healthy ear – this reflection is picked up by the machine and is termed a clear response. The operator will be able to give you the results straight away.

The majority of babies show a clear response to the first test. If they don't then further testing will be offered. A clear response may not be picked up by both ears, but this does not necessarily mean that there is a problem. There may be some fluid behind the eardrum (very common and generally temporary), or the baby may not have been completely quiet at the time of testing. In this situation you will be offered repeat testing, or a different test.

powder forms have to be combined with cooled, boiled water to create the milk.

If you do choose to bottle feed you may notice that your breasts become engorged with milk, and can be tender and uncomfortable. It can take a few days or so before your milk dries up and you return to normal. Placing a covered ice pack on your breasts, wearing a very supportive bra, tucking a chilled leaf of savoy cabbage in your bra (sounds odd but many mothers swear by it!) and taking some painkillers can help. If you change from breastfeeding to bottle feeding you could try and do it gradually so that your breasts don't become engorged. If your breasts don't appear to stop producing milk or you are very uncomfortable, visit your doctor as there are medications to help stop the production of breast milk.

'I felt under a lot of pressure to breastfeed and quite guilty when I decided to stop. It just wasn't for me. I work freelance and wasn't entitled to any maternity leave or pay and we needed the money, so by the time she was a month old I was nipping out to do jobs. I didn't get on with the breast pump so we went on to bottles. For a while I still managed to do the odd feed but my milk dried up pretty quickly. Now we bond over bottle feeding instead!' Millie, 32

DIET, EXERCISE AND SEX

A healthy diet is a lifestyle choice for always, not just for pregnancy and breastfeeding. If you are breastfeeding you will require approximately 500 extra calories per day and you may find yourself getting hungry! These extra calories should come from healthy

STOMACH EXERCISE

To help strengthen your stomach muscles, which will have been stretched during pregnancy, you can try the following exercise. Your stomach muscles are part of your core muscles involved in good posture; strengthening them will not only help you regain your figure but also help relieve and prevent backache.

- Start by lying on your back or on your side with your knees bent.
- Place your hands just below your belly button and gently breathe in.
- As you breathe out, tighten your tummy muscles by trying to pull your stomach away from your hands. This is a small movement, as if you were hollowing out your stomach. Hold it for a second.
- As you breathe in, relax your stomach muscles before repeating three times.

With time, as your muscles get stronger, you will be able to do more repetitions and hold the movement for longer (up to 10 seconds). You will also be able to do the exercise standing up. Once you have mastered this you can move on to other stomach exercises.

foods and snacks such as fresh or dried fruit, nuts and seeds, vegetables or whole grains. It is also important to keep up your fluid intake, making sure that you are drinking enough water.

Breastfeeding is not the time to put yourself on a restrictive diet in order to lose your pregnancy weight as you are producing milk and need nutrients to do so. You may wish to continue to take a vitamin supplement containing vitamin D (for more information see page 10). Breastfeeding should help you lose weight, as will a healthy diet combined with some exercise.

Initially, it can seem like you have no time for exercise as you get used to caring for your baby. However, you can start doing your pelvic floor exercises almost straight away. It is recommended that you should not embark on an intense exercise programme for approximately six weeks, or slightly longer after a Caesarean section, to allow your body time to heal. In the meantime, you can start slowly – walking while pushing your baby in a pram or buggy counts as exercise and will start to help you get back into shape. After six weeks or so you may want to join a postnatal exercise or yoga class. You can often bring your baby along to these and they are a good opportunity to meet other mums while getting fit! Exercise will also help to release endorphins and make you feel good.

You can start having sex whenever you feel ready, but it is common for both men and women to have a reduced sex drive when looking after a newborn baby. This is probably due to the combination of tiredness, changes in the dynamics of your relationship and the fact that you may have some vaginal dryness (due to hormone changes associated with breastfeeding) or soreness from an episiotomy. Many

'It was quite a while before I had the energy or even the time to have sex and I think my partner found this difficult. I tried to do other things but often I was just so exhausted that the only thing I wanted to do in bed was sleep. Thankfully my sex drive did come back. For me it was directly linked to how much sleep I got!' Lilly, 38 women are also concerned about their new body shape, or leaking or engorged breasts.

Rest assured that these feelings are common in the first few weeks and months after delivery. Make sure that you and your partner talk to each other and explain how you are feeling. You can stay physically close without sexual intercourse – even cuddling can keep you physically connected. With time, many couples find that their libido returns, though when and where you have intercourse may change when you have young children running around!

FOR FATHERS

Now is your chance to really get involved with your new baby. Even if your partner is breastfeeding there are still plenty of opportunities for you to bath the baby, change nappies, go for walks and have lots and lots of cuddles. Many fathers find it difficult to bond with their baby, or that it takes longer for them than for the mother, so the more time you spend with them, the quicker that bond will grow.

Even if you took your full two weeks of paternity allowance you will probably find that it passes extremely quickly, and before you know it you are back at work. You are probably not having as much sleep as normal so, like many new fathers, you may be feeling exhausted! Try not to get into a competition with your partner about who is the most tired, be it due to work or breastfeeding. Instead, really focus on supporting each other and remember that babies do learn to sleep with time!

Your partner will need you to help out, not just with practical things such as the washing up or shopping, but with emotional support too. Give her lots of hugs and reassure her that she is doing well. Expect her to be emotional in the first few days after birth but do watch out for the signs of postnatal depression (see page 306) as people who become depressed often find it difficult to ask for help and may need encouragement to do so. In extremely rare cases a condition called puerperal psychosis can develop where the woman starts to experience hallucinations and delusions and may lose touch with reality; in this case you would need to contact your doctor urgently.

During the first few weeks after the birth, you and your partner will both be finding your feet as parents, whether or not this is your first child. In time you will develop new roles as a family, and eventually will catch up on some sleep!

REGISTERING THE BIRTH

All babies need to be registered with the General Registry Office within 42 days (six weeks) of birth, or 21 days (three weeks) in Scotland. You will be given the information about how to register your baby while you are in hospital. Registration generally takes place in your local registry office; in some areas you need to make an appointment in advance. You will need to take with you information about your baby's date, time and place of birth, though this is generally given to you by the hospital. You will also need to know what you wish to call your baby! If you are married, both your name and your partner's name will appear on the birth certificate; if you are unmarried only your name will appear on the certificate unless the father also attends the registration. You will be given or sent a short birth certificate without charge. If you require a long certificate (which is necessary in order to apply for a passport), a small charge will be made per copy. If you do not register your child within the time limit you will be fined.

'I couldn't understand what she did all day while I was at work. How could she be so busy with just one little baby? When he was 13 weeks she went for a spa day and I was left at home with bottles for him. Suddenly I knew – it was all encompassing. I didn't even have time for a shower, never mind cooking dinner!' Tim, 37

THE SIX- TO EIGHT-WEEK BABY CHECK

The postnatal check generally occurs between six and eight weeks after delivery and can be performed by your GP or hospital doctors. It is an opportunity for both you and your baby to be checked over and to discuss any concerns you may have.

Your check will involve your doctor discussing your delivery, checking that you have recovered and asking how you are managing with your baby. Topics discussed will generally include how you are feeding the baby, how much sleep you are having, whether or not you are getting out of the house, and whether you feel supported. Your doctor may ask about your breasts if you are breastfeeding, and about any problems from any stitches or from a Caesarean. They may also ask about whether you are leaking urine and encourage you to do your pelvic floor exercises. You will be asked about your moods and how you are coping, so that they can help you if you are depressed. Contraception will also be discussed, along with any problems or concerns you may have, no matter how complicated or simple they may seem.

Your baby's check involves your doctor talking to you about any worries and a full physical examination. This is the same as the examination carried out by a paediatrician in the hospital and involves checking all the baby's systems – heart, lungs, eyes, ears, mouth, hips, limbs, genitals, tummy, reflexes and tone as well as measuring the baby's length, head circumference and weight. Your doctor will also discuss the immunisation schedule with you, informing you and answering any questions you may have about vaccines. Your baby is due the first set of immunisations when he is 8 weeks old, which can be arranged through your GP surgery.

A further aim of the postnatal check is for you to build a relationship with your GP so that you feel able to visit them with any future concerns you may have.

last word

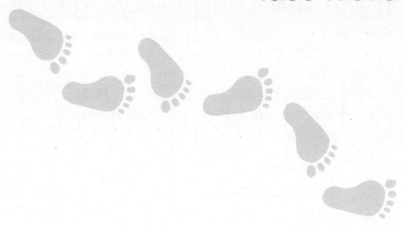

Here we are, nine months later, and you have a newborn baby. During pregnancy, with its time markings of trimesters, scans and antenatal appointments, the realities of actually having a baby can be difficult to imagine, even if you already have a child or children. It is often hard to see past pregnancy and the hurdle of labour, and suddenly – or at least it can feel quite sudden – the baby is here and the journey of pregnancy is over. But a new journey has begun – one which, as a (fairly) new mother myself, I can truthfully say is the most exciting, invigorating, terrifying and ultimately joyful adventure.

This tiny baby, who at first is not able to do anything – not even feed himself (or often not even sleep!) – is full of potential, and so are you as a parent. The excitement comes as you discover each other, become a family and learn together. Of course it can be scary, and the truth is there are no 'right' answers about parenting. Trust that you are the best mother and the best parent for your baby, and together you will work out the rest. Good luck and have fun!

appendix: pregnancy timeline

Note: these timing are approximate

1st TRIMESTER

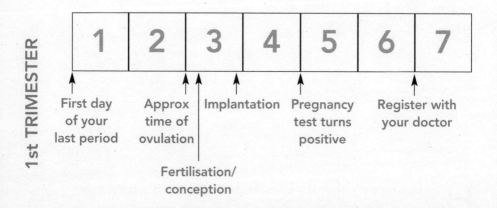

| 1 | 2 | 3 | 4 | 5 | 6 | 7 |

First day of your last period

Approx time of ovulation

Implantation

Fertilisation/ conception

Pregnancy test turns positive

Register with your doctor

2nd TRIMESTER

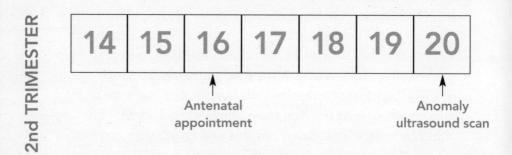

| 14 | 15 | 16 | 17 | 18 | 19 | 20 |

Antenatal appointment

Anomaly ultrasound scan

3rd TRIMESTER

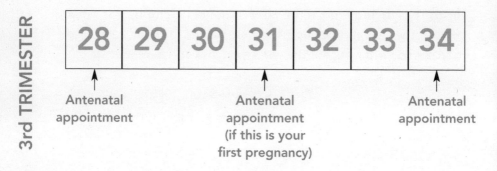

| 28 | 29 | 30 | 31 | 32 | 33 | 34 |

Antenatal appointment

Antenatal appointment (if this is your first pregnancy)

Antenatal appointment

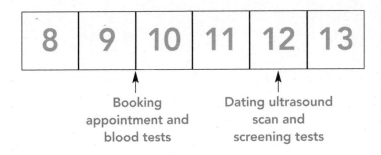

Booking
appointment and
blood tests

Dating ultrasound
scan and
screening tests

1st TRIMESTER

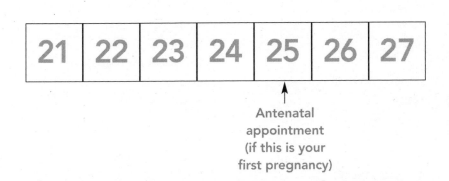

Antenatal
appointment
(if this is your
first pregnancy)

2nd TRIMESTER

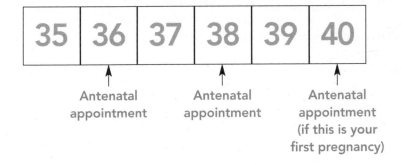

Antenatal
appointment

Antenatal
appointment

Antenatal
appointment
(if this is your
first pregnancy)

3rd TRIMESTER

323

useful addresses

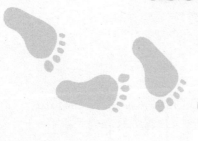

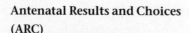

Antenatal Results and Choices (ARC)
73–75 Charlotte Street
London W1P 1LB
Tel: 020 7631 0285 (helpline)
www.arc-uk.org
Advice on antenatal tests and screening.

Association of Breastfeeding Mothers
PO Box 207
Bridgewater TA6 7YT
Tel: 08444 122 949 (helpline)
www.abm.me.uk
Provides support regarding breastfeeding.

Association for Postnatal Illness
154 Dawes Road
London SW6 7EB
Tel: 020 7386 0868
www.apni.org
Provides support for mothers with postnatal illness.

Breastfeeding Network
PO Box 1126
Paisley PA2 8YB
Tel: 0870 900 8787 (helpline)
www.breastfeedingnetwork.org.uk
Provides information and support regarding breastfeeding.

Department for Work and Pensions
www.dwp.gov.uk

Directgov
www.direct.gov.uk

HM Revenue & Customs
www.hmrc.gov.uk
Information on maternity and paternity rights, leave, pay and other issues.

Eating for Pregnancy
www.eatingforpregnancy.co.uk
Gives information regarding healthy and safe eating in pregnancy.

Gingerbread/One Parent Families
225 Kentish Town Road
London NW5 2LX
Tel: 020 7428 5400
Tel: 0800 018 5026 (helpline)
www.gingerbread.org.uk
www.oneparentfamily.co.uk
Gives information regarding local support and self-help groups for single parents.

Home-Start
Tel: 0800 068 6368 (free information line)
www.home-start.org.uk
Charitable organisation providing support and friendship for parents of children under five.

Independent Midwives' Association
1 The Great Quarry
Guildford
Surrey GU1 3XN
Tel: 01483 821104
www.independentmidwives.org.uk

La Leche League
PO Box 29
West Bridgford
Nottingham NG2 7NP
Tel: 0845 120 2918 (helpline)
www.laleche.org.uk
Gives support and advice regarding breastfeeding.

Maternity Action
The Grayston Centre
28 Charles Square
London N1 6HT
www.maternityaction.org.uk
Promotes the wellbeing of parents, mothers-to-be and children and challenges inequality.

Meet-A-Mum Association (MAMA)
Tel: 0845 120 3746 (helpline; 7pm–10pm Monday to Friday only)
www.mama.co.uk
Provides support and friendship for mothers and mothers-to-be.

The Miscarriage Association
c/o Clayton Hospital
Northgate
Wakefield WF1 3JS
Tel: 01924 200799 (helpline; 9am–4pm Monday to Friday)
www.miscarriageassociation.org.uk
Provides support and information for those who have lost a pregnancy.

National Childbirth Trust
Alexandra House
Oldham Terrace
London W3 6NH
Tel: 0870 444 9709 (pregnancy and
birth information line)
Tel: 0870 444 8708 (breastfeeding
helpline)
Tel: 0300 33 00 770 (enquiries)
www.nct.org.uk
*Support and information regarding
pregnancy, childbirth and early
parenthood. Gives information
regarding local antenatal and
postnatal classes and nearly new sales.*

NHS Direct
Tel: 0845 46 47
www.nhsdirect.nhs.uk
Advice regarding health matters.

Parentline Plus
520 Highgate Studios
53–79 Highgate Road
Kentish Town
London NW5 1TL
Tel: 020 7284 5500
Tel: 0808 800 2222 (helpline)
www.parentlineplus.org.uk
*Information and support for families;
phone support, email support and
parenting groups.*

Quit
211 Old Street
London EC1V 9NR
Tel: 020 7251 1551

Tel: 0800 002200
(Quitline/helpline)
NHS pregnancy smoking helpline:
0800 169 9 169 (free one-to-one
counselling and support)
www.quit.org.uk
*Charity to provide support and help to
stop smoking.*

**Royal College of Obstetricians
and Gynaecologists**
www.rcog.org.uk
*The website has patient information
leaflets on various topics within
pregnancy.*

**Twins and Multiple Birth
Association (TAMBA)**
2 The Willows
Gardner Road
Guildford
Surrey GU1 4PG
Tel: 0800 138 0509 (helpline)
Tel: 01483 304 442
www.tamba.org.uk
*Charity providing support and
information for families with twins,
triplets or more.*

Working Families
1–3 Berry Street
London EC1V 0AA
Tel: 020 7253 7243
www.workingfamilies.org.uk
*Information and support about
working life with a family.*

glossary

Amniocentesis: a test performed by removing some amniotic fluid to test for certain genetic or chromosomal disorders.

Amniotic fluid: the fluid within the amniotic membrane surrounding the foetus.

Amniotic membrane (amnion): a membrane that surrounds the fluid and foetus in the womb.

Anomaly scan: ultrasound scan carried out at approximately 20 weeks to check the baby's major organs, head and limbs.

Antenatal: literally 'before birth' – the time before giving birth, that is, pregnancy.

Anterior position: where the baby is head down with his face towards the mother's back – the optimum position for delivery.

Anti-D: an injection of immunoglobulin given to all women who have the blood group Rhesus negative at various stages during pregnancy and after labour to prevent the body building up potentially harmful antibodies against the foetus.

Areola: the area of coloured skin around the nipple.

Blastocyst: a very early stage of development of the embryo.

Booking appointment: the first appointment with a midwife when a full history and various blood tests will be taken.

Braxton Hicks contractions: 'practice' contractions that often feel like a tightening sensation in the womb.

Breech: in a breech presentation the baby is not head down; rather the part nearest the mother's pelvis is his bottom or feet.

Caesarean section: an operation to deliver the baby.

Cephalic: the baby is facing head down in the pelvis.

Cervix: the neck of the womb.

Chorionic villous sampling (CVS): a test to check for chromosomal conditions in the foetus, performed by obtaining a sample of the placenta.

Chromosome: structure within a cell that contains genetic information.

Colostrum: the first milk, or pre-milk, which is secreted in the first few days after delivery. It is rich in antibodies and gradually changes to mature milk.

Combined test: a test combining blood tests and a measurement on ultrasound to screen for various conditions.

Conception: when a sperm fertilises an egg.

Contractions: regular tightenings of the womb to dilate the cervix and push the baby out during labour.

Crowning: the moment in labour when the baby's head becomes and stays visible without slipping back into the birth canal between contractions.

Dating scan: generally the first ultrasound scan in pregnancy, at around 12 weeks, when the estimated delivery date is calculated.

Dilation/dilatation: the opening or widening of the cervix in labour.

Electronic foetal monitoring: a method of monitoring the baby during the later stages of pregnancy or during labour, using pads and a machine to pick up the baby's heartbeat.

Embryo: the medical term for the developing baby up until the eighth week of pregnancy.

Engaged: the baby's head has dropped into the pelvis.

Entonox: (see gas and air)

Epidural: a method of pain relief during labour in which anaesthetic is inserted into the lower spine.

Episiotomy: a small cut into the perineum (area between the vagina and anus) to help the baby be delivered.

Expected delivery date (EDD): the expected date on which the baby will be born, calculated from the date of the last period or from the dating scan.

External cephalic version (ECV): a procedure to try and turn a breech baby into a head-down position by manipulating it through the abdomen.

Fertilisation: when a sperm fuses with an egg.

Foetus: the medical term for the developing baby from eight weeks' gestation until it is born.

Forceps: a surgical tool that fits round the baby's head to help guide it through the birth canal.

Gas and air (also called Entonox): a mixture of gases that can be used for pain relief during labour.

Gene: found on chromosomes; carries inherited material.

Gestation: the period from fertilisation to delivery, that is, pregnancy. How many weeks' gestation you are is the same as how many weeks pregnant you are.

Gestational diabetes: a form of diabetes that develops in pregnancy and generally resolves after the baby is born.

Glucose tolerance test: a test carried out, generally at around 28 weeks' gestation, involving blood tests and drinking a sugary drink to see if the mother has developed gestational diabetes.

Haemoglobin: a structure in red blood cells which carries oxygen around the body.

Haemorrhage: excessive bleeding.

HCG (human chorionic gonadotrophin): a hormone produced by the placenta; sometimes called 'pregnancy hormone' as it is the hormone picked up on a pregnancy test.

Hyperemesis gravidarum: severe and excessive vomiting in pregnancy resulting in dehydration.

Implantation: when the early embryo attaches itself to the lining of the womb. The site at which this happens determines the site of the placenta.

Induction: when labour is started artificially.

Labour: the process in which the baby and placenta are delivered. It can also be used to mean hard physical work, which labour is!

LMP (last menstrual period): the first day of the last period, used to calculate the expected delivery date.

Maternity leave: time off work to look after a baby.

Maternity pay: wages during maternity leave.

Meconium: the contents of the baby's intestines, which come out as the first sticky and dark green stool.

Menstrual cycle: the cycle in which a woman produces an egg, the lining of the womb prepares itself for implantation and is then shed as a period if pregnancy does not occur.

Midwife: the person who cares for a woman during pregnancy and labour.

Miscarriage: pregnancy loss before 24 weeks' gestation.

Mucus plug: a small plug of mucus in the cervix that protects the baby from infection. This comes out in the 'show'.

Obstetrician: a doctor who specialises in the care of pregnant women.

Oedema: accumulation of excessive fluid in the body, causing puffiness.

Oestrogen: a hormone with many roles, including the development of breasts and increasing blood flow to the mother's organs.

Ovulation: the point at which an egg is released from the ovary to be picked up by the fallopian tube.

Ovum: an egg; the sex cell of the woman which is released every month during the menstrual cycle.

Oxytocin: a hormone produced by the brain that stimulates the womb to contract in labour, as well as the production of breast milk.

Pelvic floor: a collection of muscles in the pelvis that support your bladder and womb.

Perineum: area of skin and soft tissue between the anus and vagina.

Pethidine: a painkilling drug that can be given by injection during labour.

Placenta: an organ attached to the lining of the womb; it has a role in supplying oxygen and glucose to the baby while getting rid of any waste products.

Placenta praevia: a low-lying placenta, which may cover the cervix.

Posterior position: when the baby is head down but facing the mother's tummy, so his back is facing her back.

Postnatal: after a woman has given birth.

Postpartum period: the six weeks after a woman has given birth.

Pre-eclampsia: a condition of pregnancy characterised by high blood pressure, protein in the urine and oedema (fluid retention). Can lead to eclampsia.

Premature/preterm: a baby born before 37 weeks' gestation.

Prenatal: (see antenatal)

Progesterone: a hormone with many roles including relaxing the muscles of your digestive tract and dilating your blood vessels.

Quickening: the first time a woman feels her baby move.

Show: when the cervical mucus plug comes away.

Sperm: the male sex cell, found in semen, which fertilises an egg.

Station: a measure of how far the baby's head or presenting part has descended into the pelvis.

Symphysis fundal height: the measurement between the top of the uterus (fundus) and pubic bone, taken at antenatal appointments; correlates roughly to how many weeks pregnant a woman is.

Syntocinon: an artificial version of the hormone oxytocin, used to induce or speed up labour.

Trimester: pregnancy is divided into three periods called trimesters. Generally Weeks 1–13 make up the first trimester, 13–26 the second, and 27–40 the third, though there is some disagreement about the exact start and end dates of each trimester.

Ultrasound scan: a method of visualising the baby using very high-frequency sound waves. In pregnancy, women are generally offered two scans – the dating scan at around 12 weeks and the anomaly scan at around 20 weeks.

Umbilical cord: cord connecting the baby to the placenta.

Uterus: womb, the part of your body in which the baby develops.

Ventouse: a small cup is attached to the baby's head and suction used to help guide it out through the birth canal.

Waters breaking: when the amniotic membranes rupture and the amniotic fluid leaks out.

Womb: (see uterus)

Zygote: the medical term for an egg that has been fertilised by a sperm.

index

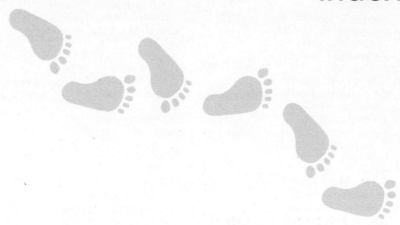

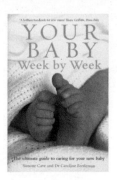